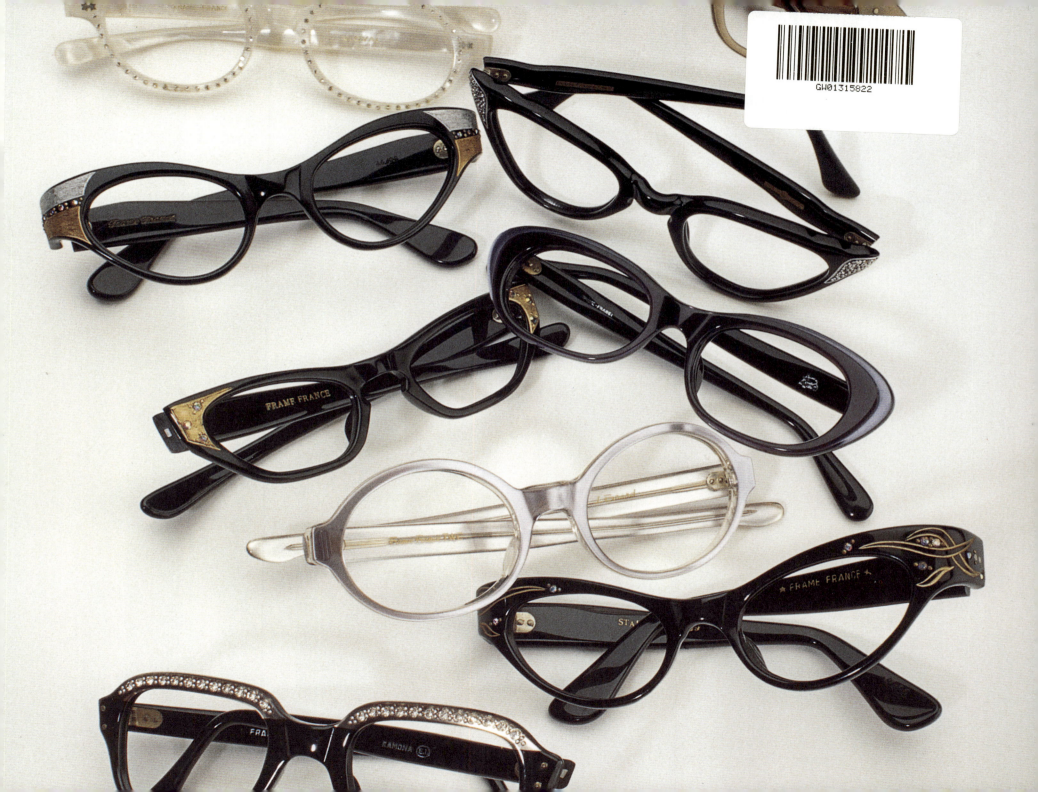

EYEGLASS
RETROSPECTIVE

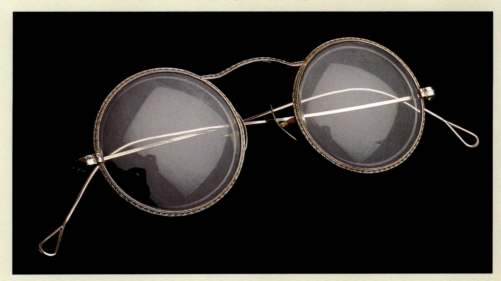

WHERE FASHION MEETS SCIENCE

NANCY N. SCHIFFER

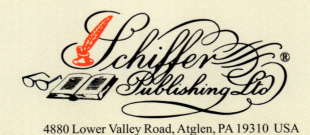

4880 Lower Valley Road, Atglen, PA 19310 USA

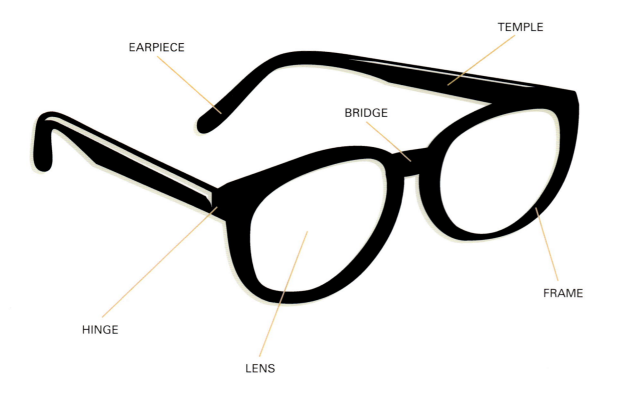

Schiffer, Nancy.
  Eyeglass retrospective: where fashion meets science / Nancy N. Schiffer.
    p. cm.
  Includes bibliographical references and index.
  ISBN 0-7643-1041-0 (hardcover)
  1. Eyeglasses--History. I. Title.
  GT2370.S35 2000
  391.4'4--dc21   99-050076

Copyright © 2000 by Nancy N. Schiffer

All rights reserved. No part of this work may be reproduced or used in any form or by any means—graphic, electronic, or mechanical, including photocopying or information storage and retrieval systems—without written permission from the copyright holder.
"Schiffer," "Schiffer Publishing Ltd. & Design," and the "Design of pen and inkwell" are registered trademarks of Schiffer Publishing Ltd.

Cover design by Bruce Waters
Book design by Blair Loughrey
Type set in Zurich (variation) / Goudy Olst Bt
ISBN: 0-7643-1041-0
Printed in China
1 2 3 4

Published by Schiffer Publishing Ltd.
4880 Lower Valley Road
Atglen, PA 19310
Phone: (610) 593-1777; Fax: (610) 593-2002
E-mail: Schifferbk@aol.com
Please visit our web site catalog at
www.schifferbooks.com
Please write for a free catalog.
This book may be purchased from the publisher.
Please include $3.95 for shipping.

In Europe, Schiffer books are distributed by
Bushwood Books
6 Marksbury Ave.
Kew Gardens
Surrey TW9 4JF England
Phone: 44 (0)208-392-8585; Fax: 44 (0)208-392-9876
E-mail: Bushwd@aol.com
Free postage in the UK. Europe: air mail at cost.
Please try your bookstore first.

We are interested in hearing from authors with book ideas on related subjects.

Back cover: Courtesy of Mercurá, NYC.

CONTENTS

ACKNOWLEDGEMENTS	**4**
PREFACE	**5**
EARLIEST EYEWEAR	**7**
EUROPEAN STYLES	**8**
CHINESE STYLES	**12**
18TH CENTURY	**17**
19TH CENTURY	**27**
MCALLISTER OPTICIANS	**40**
LORGNETTES	**51**
PINCE-NEZ	**60**
SPECIALIZED GLASSES	**64**
20TH CENTURY	**69**
BIBLIOGRAPHY	**191**
INDEX	**191**

ACKNOWLEDGEMENTS

Looking back at the process of compiling this book includes a grateful glance at many people who contributed their time, effort, and deep personal knowledge of eyewear. They each have helped me to recognize scientific developments and visualize evolving fashions. Each, therefore, has illuminated my initial interest and opened my eyes to eyewear's development. I look forward to many future conversations with them about discoveries, insights, and trends. My gratitude goes specifically to Dee Battle, Mary Ann Berlangieri, Barbara Blau, Alfonso Carnuccio, Doug Congdon-Martin, Bill Drucker, Helene Fendelman, Mallory Gerber, A. Oliver Goldsmith, Pamela Gorenflo, Aida Guzzi, John Handley, Victoria Hansen, Molly Higgins, John Rice Irwin, Charles E. Letocha, Bob Lyons, Desire Smith, Brian Stewart, John and Valda Tull, Licia A. Wells, and Mike Wilson. I also thank my photographers, Blair Loughrey, Jeff Snyder, and Bruce Waters, whose sharp eyes behind the camera lens lets us all see the subject more clearly.

PREFACE

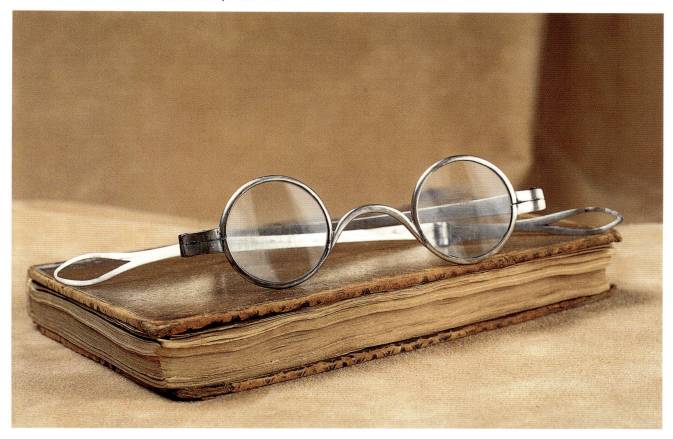

Steel frames with folding temples and looped ends, not marked. Oliver Goldsmith Eyewear Ltd.

Sometimes we fail to see what is right before our eyes. My interest in eyewear grows out of many years studying popular decorative arts including the furniture, ceramics, toys, and jewelry with which each generation defines itself. It is interesting to notice how we can look at an image (painting, drawing, photograph) and determine pretty accurately what era it depicts through the designs of the artifacts represented. Clues include the popular arts and certainly extend to eyewear—which has been so taken for granted as to be overlooked. But if we open our minds and eyes, we can see eyewear as it truly appears today, as a bridge between fashion and science.

MATERIALS

As scientific knowledge advanced through the centuries, new materials were employed to meet the demand for better eyewear- for vision aids first, and then for fashion. When I noticed sunglasses that are made today with newly-developed materials being worn by style-conscious individuals, I wondered through what development have they come to their current popularity?

DESIGNS

As scientific facts about vision became better understood over the centuries, better lenses were made to improve the wearer's sight. The designs of frames were changed as more comfortable and practical styles were invented. In the mid-twentieth century, eyeglass makers carefully sought high profile movie stars and music entertainers to wear their designs in order to promote their companies. Advertising worked its magic and the general public came to prefer the advertised designs. How did this happen?

STATUS SYMBOLS

As the history of eyewear was studied, certain trends were found to be repeated. In former times, people with poor vision apologized for having to put on glasses to read a document. Funny to me was the realization that in China, eyeglasses have been not only vision aids but also status symbols associated with scholars and learned people. In the nineteenth century in the West, the wearing of a monocle was probably a fashion affectation. Correlations today are seen as many people who have perfectly fine natural vision wear sunglasses day and night to project an appealing image. Why did this happen?

With these questions in mind, the search for their answers was sought by looking carefully at the evidence that existing eyewear, both old and contemporary, puts right before our eyes. How the evidence is interpreted will determine the answers. This book attempts to share the findings and provide an overview for identifying and dating eyewear that can be found on the market today.

EVALUATING EYEGLASSES

Eyeglasses and their cases are found in antiques markets worldwide for a wide range of values depending on their condition, age, materials, history, rarity, and location of the market. City prices are usually more than country prices. We have included the prices of items that were available for purchase at the time this book was written as a courtesy to those who want this factual information as a guide. Of course, being at the right place with knowledge at the right time can make a big difference. We hope to offer some of the knowledge necessary to make an educated offer.

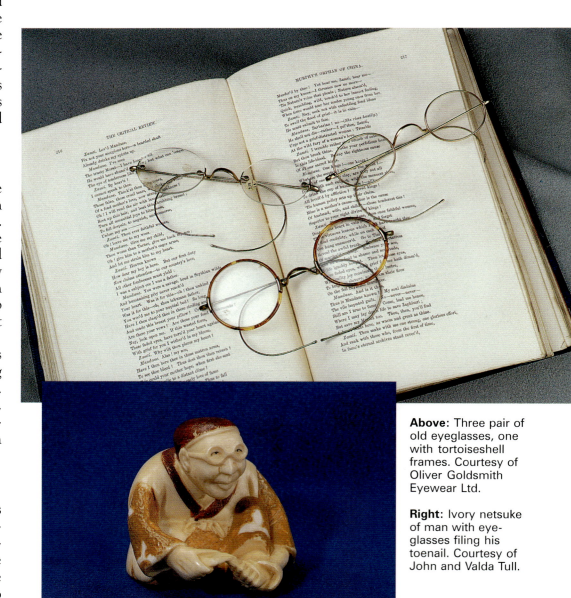

Above: Three pair of old eyeglasses, one with tortoiseshell frames. Courtesy of Oliver Goldsmith Eyewear Ltd.

Right: Ivory netsuke of man with eyeglasses filing his toenail. Courtesy of John and Valda Tull.

EARLIEST EYEWEAR

The need for protection from exposure surely caused primitive man to shield his eyes from the sun and wind in his earliest days of existence. Eskimo shades are too old to have a history, and they certainly are necessities in the present arctic regions.

It is not definitely known when or where the first eyeglasses, as we know them today, were invented. However, the year 1287 and northern Italy has been suggested because of various technologies that made their construction possible, and drawn representations of people with them, that date from this time and locale.

The ancient Chinese are credited with inventing glass. Chinese eyeglasses are shown in Medieval drawings, but were they brought to or from China by early Spanish missionaries?

Definitive answers have not been given to such questions, and probably cannot be, with present knowledge. It is well beyond the scope of this study to determine when eyeglasses first appeared and whether they originated in Europe or China. Scholars have studied evidence and continue to search for indications to confirm the roots of the forms, and it is fascinating to follow their thoughts through existing materials. Interested readers are encouraged to consult the bibliography where readily accessible references containing the opinions of many authors regarding these questions are found. Richard Corson particularly has gathered illustrations and literary references from early sources in his book. Scholarly and scientific articles are heavily quoted in J. William Rosenthal's book.

Above: Photograph of Eskimo man with snow goggles. Courtesy of John and Valda Tull

Left: Eskimo snow goggles made from bone, baleen, and wood. Courtesy of John and Valda Tull

EUROPEAN STYLES

Throughout the Middle Ages in Europe, religious monasteries were the only sanctuaries of knowledge and learning. There, ideas were preserved by being written down and copied by handwriting alone. No vision aids are thought to have been available to the writers of Medieval manuscripts, and so their careers were probably over by the age of forty.

By the 13th century, enough of a glass industry existed in Venice, Italy, for the possibility of flat glass to be made there. Illustrations of that time depict the first pictures showing people, religious leaders in fact, with vision aids. Analysis of the pictures, their social periods, and current technical knowledge suggests that in the area of northern Italy eyeglasses in an early form could have been invented. Spanish, Italian, and other traders of the 14th and 15th centuries traveled to Asia. Could they have taken eyeglasses of some sort along with them as trade items?

In Europe, the trail of eyeglasses can be tracked through illustrations and literature from the 14th century forward. Terminology referring to eyeglasses made its way into languages from early times. For example, colored lenses appeared very early: in German the term for eyeglasses, *brille*, probably comes from the gemstone beryl [green beryl is emerald] from which some lenses are believed to have been made. As mechanical printing methods evolved, and after moveable type was invented in Mainz, Germany, by printer Johannes Gutenberg about 1450, more words could be read by more people, and a general need for inexpensive vision aids gradually developed.

Nuremberg Magnifiers

A small industry grew up in Nuremberg (south German region) to make magnifying glasses, and by the 17th century they produced single, round, glass lens magnifiers, usually bound with a metal frame and handle, in significant numbers. The Nuremberg magnifiers were sold with papier maché or wooden cases, and occasionally can be found to this day.

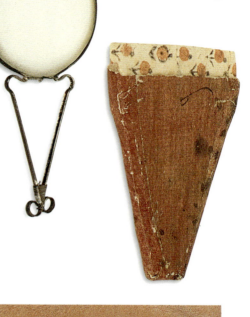

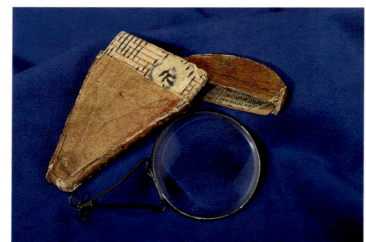

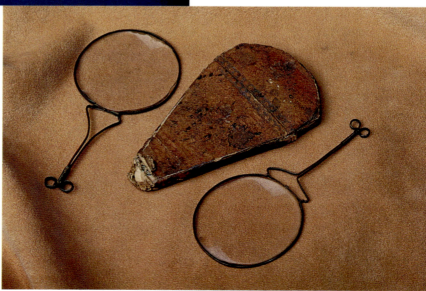

Top right: Magnifying glass, Germany, c. 1750-1800. Glass, metal, paper. Courtesy of The Museum of Ophthalmology, Foundation of the American Academy of Ophthalmology, San Francisco.

Above: Nuremberg magnifying glass in papier maché case. Courtesy of John and Valda Tull.

Right: Nuremberg magnifying glasses and papier maché case with sliding lid.

Eyeglasses

Evidence of eyeglasses with two joined frames being readily available to the European public in the seventeenth century is frequent. Street vendors of small articles, including spectacles, is well documented in literature and pictures. The Dutch tiles shown date from the early seventeenth century and show vendors with spectacles whose precise forms and materials, of course, only can be speculated.

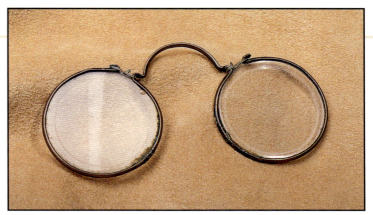

Above: Very old glasses with grinding marks on the lenses and simple frames bound at the tops with metal wire.

Right & below: Two Delft tiles, c. 1640, showing spectacles vendor.

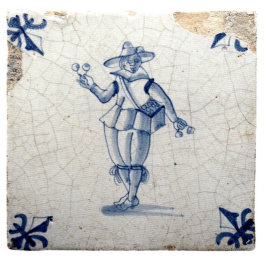

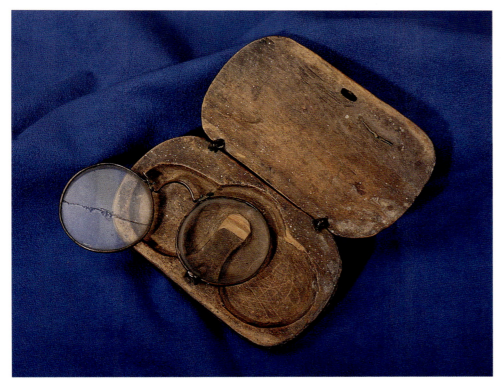

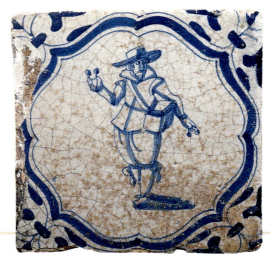

Pair of pince-nez glasses marked around the frames Johan Erhard, with beveled glass lenses, in hinged wooden case marked MP. Courtesy of John and Valda Tull.

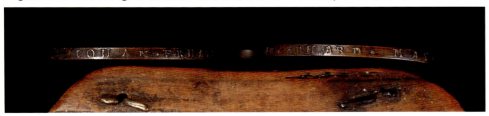

Leather Frames

Eyeglasses with two lenses and leather frames predate the eighteenth century and were probably made by shoemakers who had the knowledge, tools, and materials readily available. Leather-framed eyeglasses belonged to common people who needed visual correction; they are not beautiful or fashionable, only useful. Dating an extant pair is difficult because leather apparently was in use as eyeglass frames for several centuries and because so few have survived to the present. They are extremely rare and valuable today. The examples shown display variations in frame widths and bridge shapes.

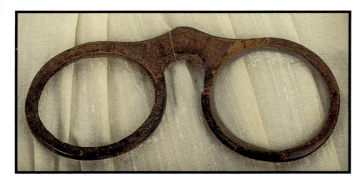

Above: Spectacles. Glass, leather. Possibly German, c. before 1700. Courtesy of The Museum of Ophthalmology, Foundation of the American Academy of Ophthalmology, San Francisco.

Right: Three pair of leather framed eyeglasses, c. before 1700, each with glass lenses.

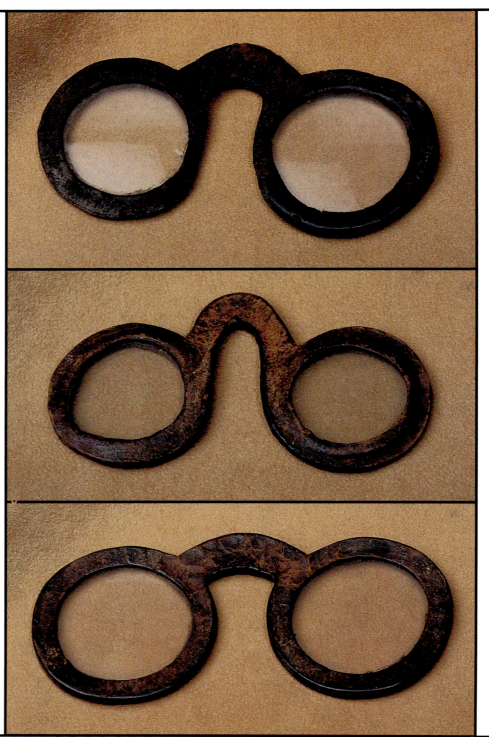

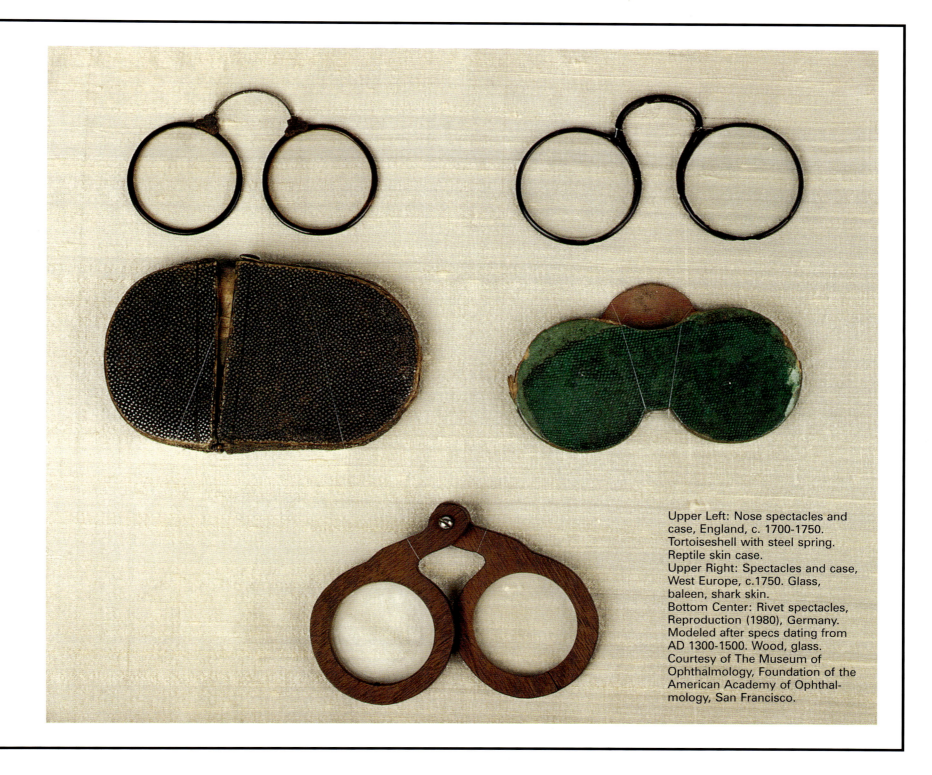

Upper Left: Nose spectacles and case, England, c. 1700-1750. Tortoiseshell with steel spring. Reptile skin case.
Upper Right: Spectacles and case, West Europe, c.1750. Glass, baleen, shark skin.
Bottom Center: Rivet spectacles, Reproduction (1980), Germany. Modeled after specs dating from AD 1300-1500. Wood, glass. Courtesy of The Museum of Ophthalmology, Foundation of the American Academy of Ophthalmology, San Francisco.

CHINESE STYLES

While their relative age, uses, and claims of originality are subjects of debate, old Chinese spectacles are distinctive in design from Western styles. Here Chinese examples are presented for comparison with Western styles and so that they can be identified; they are available in the marketplace and should be correctly recognized.

The lenses of pre-nineteenth century Chinese spectacles are usually round and may be either rimless or surrounded with a frame. While the majority of lenses, either unground or ground, are glass, they also may be clear or tea-colored quartz (tea-stone [*ai tai*]) or mica in light or dark shades.

The frames, whether folding or straight, can be found in many materials and combinations, including brass, bronze, silver, tortoiseshell, horn, lacquer, and reed. Styles before the 18th century had no side pieces but were held onto the face by looped strings which ran through two small holes in the frame at the outside of each lens and around the wearer's ears. Various methods of attaching Chinese spectacles to the face from the 18th century on can be found, including short and folding temples, loops of string, and strings with weights. Many Chinese frames have rectangular and/or pierced tortoiseshell nose pieces (bridges), distinctive to Chinese styles and in contrast with Western curved bridges.

Some writers relate that ancient Chinese people wore spectacles for purposes other than improving sight. Some people believed the lens materials themselves had healing benefits, and the eyeglasses' association with the few scholars and important people who read documents made them icons of high rank. Generally, spectacles were expensive in China at all times, and so they may have become a status item which was worn merely to demonstrate high social position. Their actual benefits to vision seem to have been sometimes unimportant.

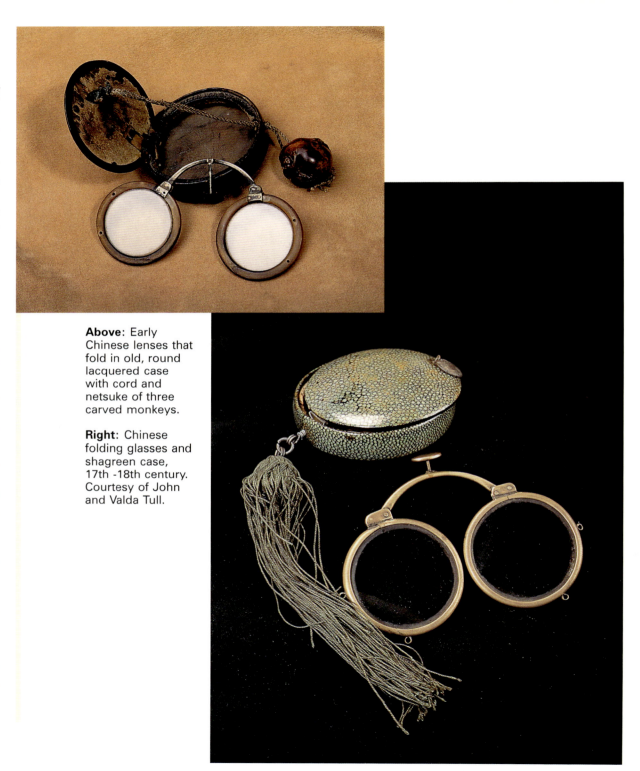

Above: Early Chinese lenses that fold in old, round lacquered case with cord and netsuke of three carved monkeys.

Right: Chinese folding glasses and shagreen case, 17th -18th century. Courtesy of John and Valda Tull.

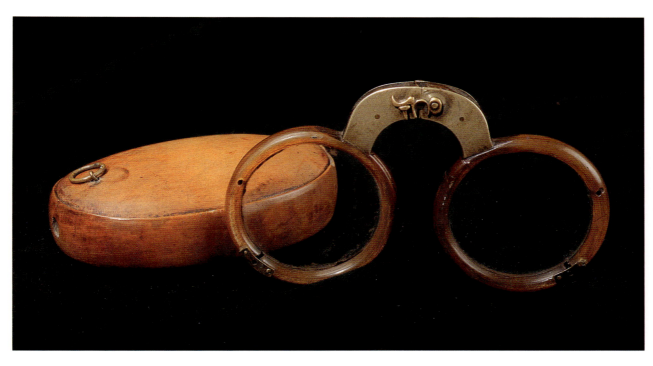

Left: Chinese wooden case made for the accompanying hinged spectacles, 17th-18th century. Courtesy of John and Valda Tull.

Below: Spectacles of brass and tortoiseshell and case of lizard skin and metal. China, 1750. Courtesy of The Museum of Ophthalmology, Foundation of the American Academy of Ophthalmology, San Francisco.

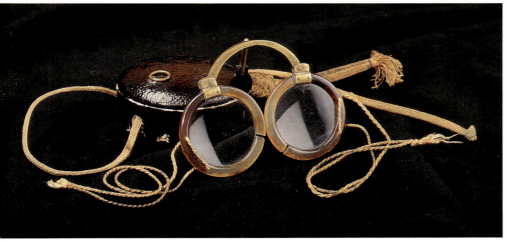

Chinese folding glasses and case, 17th-18th century. Courtesy of John and Valda Tull.

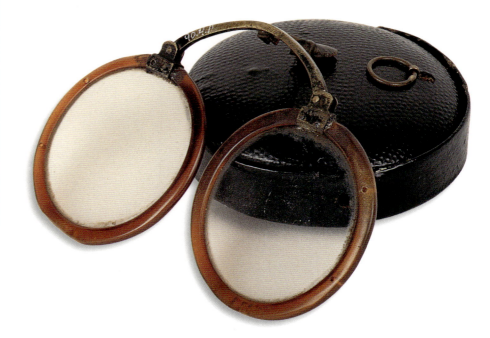

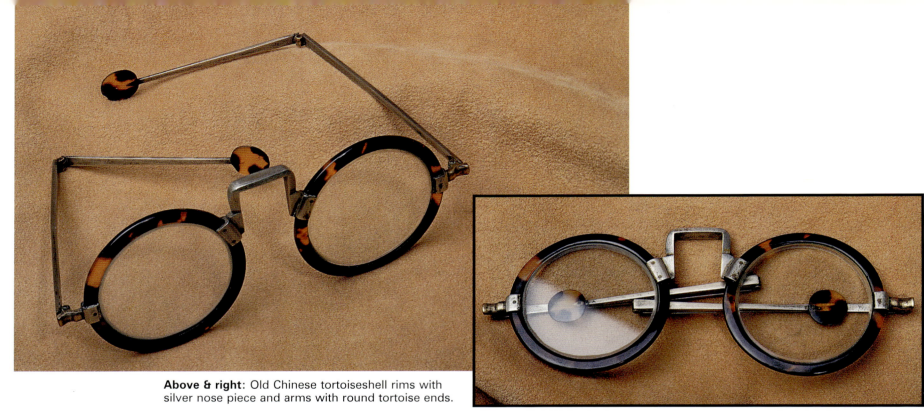

Above & right: Old Chinese tortoiseshell rims with silver nose piece and arms with round tortoise ends.

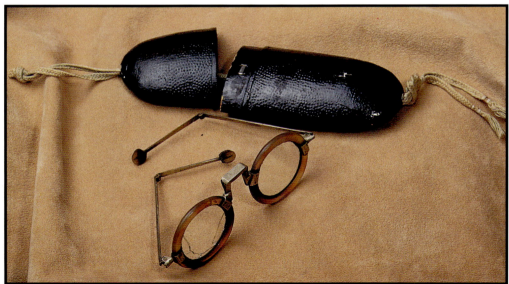

Old Chinese horn rims with silver nose piece, hinges and arms, and 2-part lacquered case with cord closure.

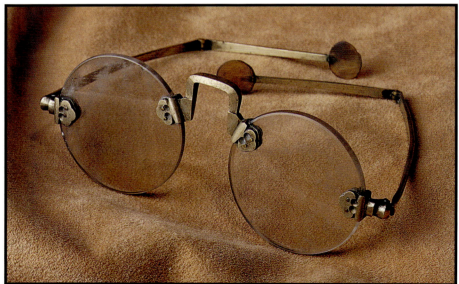

Large Chinese silver frames and quartz lenses with no power, hinged arms.

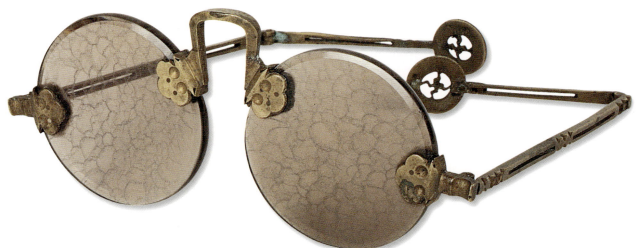

Spectacles. Tortoiseshell, brass, ai-tai (quartz). China, c. 1750. Courtesy of The Museum of Ophthalmology, Foundation of the American Academy of Ophthalmology, San Francisco.

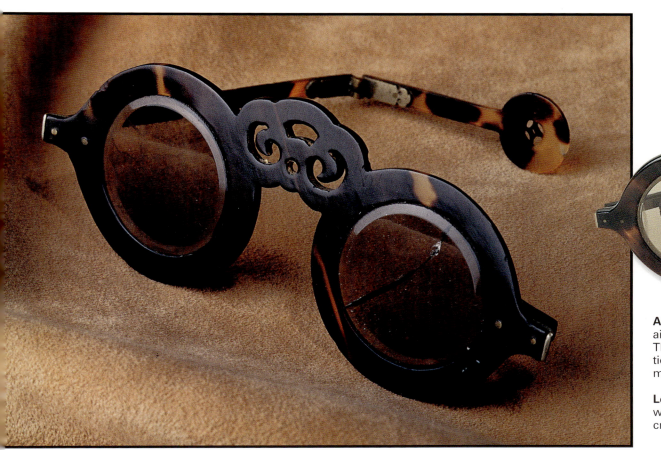

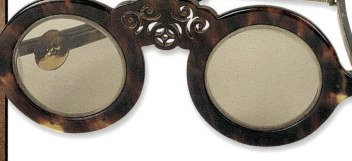

Above: Spectacles. Tortoiseshell, brass, ai-tai (quartz). China, 1750. Courtesy of The Museum of Ophthalmology, Foundation of the American Academy of Ophthalmology, San Francisco.

Left: Old Chinese tortoiseshell frames with carved bridge, one tinted lens cracked, no power in the lenses.

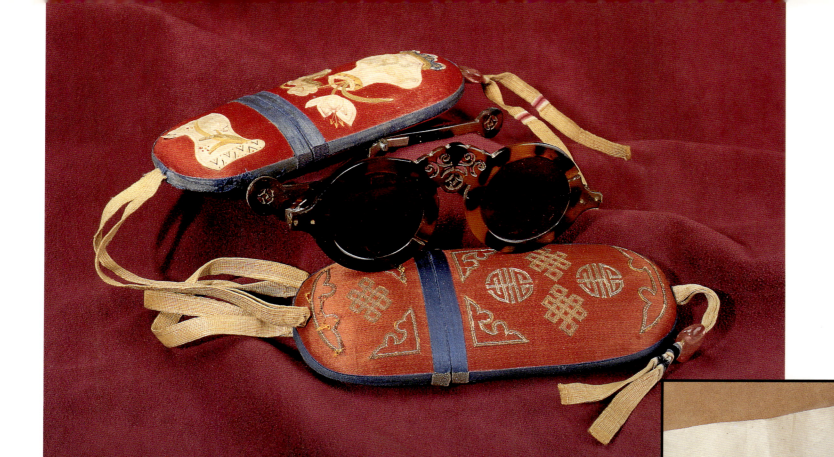

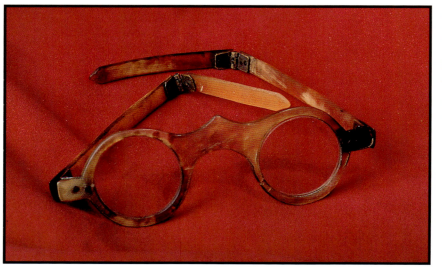

Above: Chinese glasses and embroidered cases, early 19th century. Courtesy of John and Valda Tull

Left: Horn pair with folding temple pieces and round lenses.

Right: Modern reproduction Chinese glasses from mainland China, 1988.

18TH CENTURY

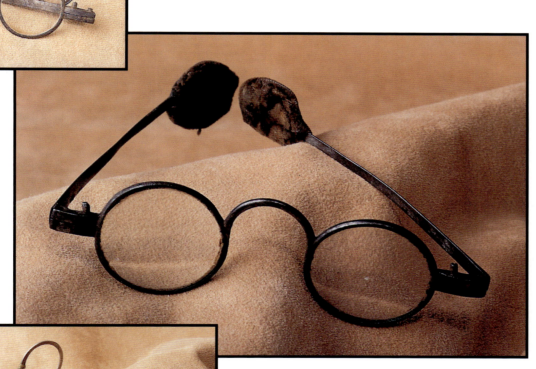

Top: Steel eyeglasses with very wide bridge and straight temples ending in large circles.

Center: Steel eyeglasses with pads on the temple piece ends.

Bottom: Silver frames with green glass for reading (easy on the eyes) and short temples.

Temple Spectacles

Previous to the 18th century, eyeglasses consisted of round, single lens glass magnifiers [see section] or double lenses. The double style consisted of two singles mounted in frames that were hand held [lorgnette, see section] or propped upon the nose [as with the leather ones shown].

A better way to hold eyeglasses in place developed about 1730 by the addition of short, stiff, hinged side pieces that clung to the wearer's temples. The side pieces are usually called "temples." Eyeglasses with this design are known in the terminology of their day as "temple spectacles." This design was a breakthrough which has been retained up to the present day.

The earliest temple pieces were short to fit under wigs and ended in rings; they were sometimes made more comfortable when the rings were padded with fabric. The temple pieces were attached at the outside edges of frames for round lenses with projecting hinges. As the century progressed, the temple

Spectacles. Iron, glass. c. 1740-1750, with hinged temples. Courtesy of The Museum of Ophthalmology, Foundation of the American Academy of Ophthalmology, San Francisco.

Colored glass in spectacles. Iron, glass, fabric. c. 1750. The green glass lenses Courtesy of The Museum of Ophthalmology, Foundation of the American Academy of Ophthalmology, San Francisco.

pieces were sometimes made longer and with turnpin hinges so they could be worn either short with a wig or long to fit at the ears. Double-hinged extensions were advertised by James Ayscough of England in 1752.

By the last quarter of the eighteenth century, glass lenses, both clear and colored, were hand-made and shaped smaller and oval as well as round. Addison Smith was granted the first English patent (No. 1389) for eyeglasses in 1783 for his design with hinged double lenses.

Eyeglass frames were generally hand-made from steel in the late 18th century. English and European eyeglasses of this period generally have c-curved steel around the bridge of the nose. French glasses of the mid-century also show x- and k-shaped bridges in steel. Silver frames became available in mid-century, but they were very expensive and not plentiful. Other frame materials used in this period include gold, brass, and horn.

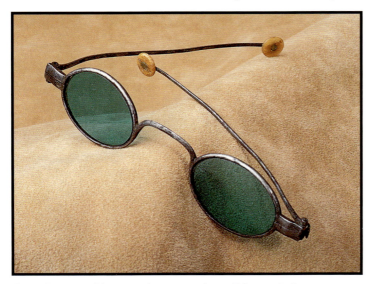

Steel frames with green lenses and small horn circles at the temples, probably for added comfort.

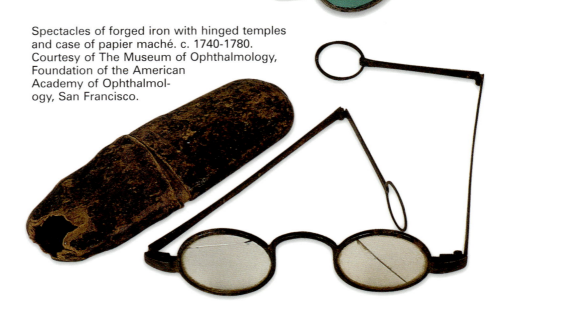

Spectacles of forged iron with hinged temples and case of papier maché. c. 1740-1780. Courtesy of The Museum of Ophthalmology, Foundation of the American Academy of Ophthalmology, San Francisco.

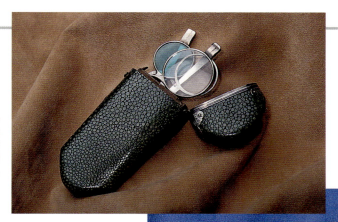

Two pair of eyeglasses within a shagreen case, silver frames, green and clear glass lenses.

Cases

The cases for eyeglasses of this period were made from paper, leather, or wood, plain or covered with sharkskin (called shagreen). Simple styles had flap or sliding openings while more elaborate styles of cases could have metal trim and hinges. In mid-century tortoiseshell cases appeared for wealthy customers and these proved durable; many have survived to the present.

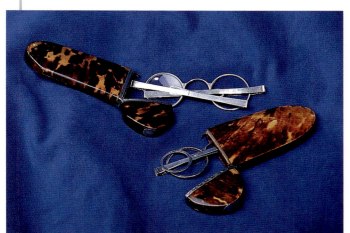

Two pair of eyeglasses in tortoiseshell cases.

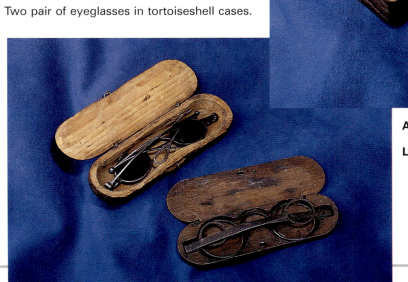

Above: Two pair of eyeglasses in wooden cases.

Left: Two pair of eyeglasses in wooden cases.

Martin's Margins

Benjamin Martin (1704-1782), an English optician, designed a new style of eyeglass frames in 1756. His new design, which has become known as Martin's Margins and is so-called to this day, has a circular obstruction around violet colored, round, biconvex lenses which are tilted inward within a steel or silver frame. The obstruction, found in various widths, is usually formed from horn or tortoiseshell. Martin's design apparently sold well, but has not had lasting influence on the design of eyeglasses thereafter.

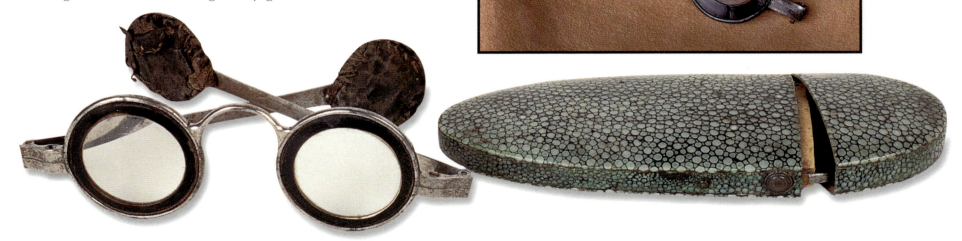

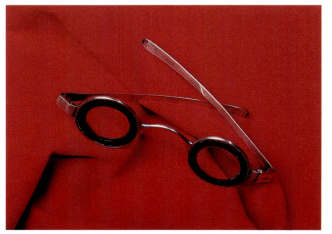

Top: Two Martin's Margins eyeglasses, c. 1760-1790, for cataract patients, they cut down light, with steel arms.

Above: Martin's Margins eyeglasses and case, England, c. 1760. Steel. Sharkskin case. Courtesy of The Museum of Ophthalmology, Foundation of the American Academy of Ophthalmology, San Francisco.

Left: Martin's Margins with silver ear pieces.

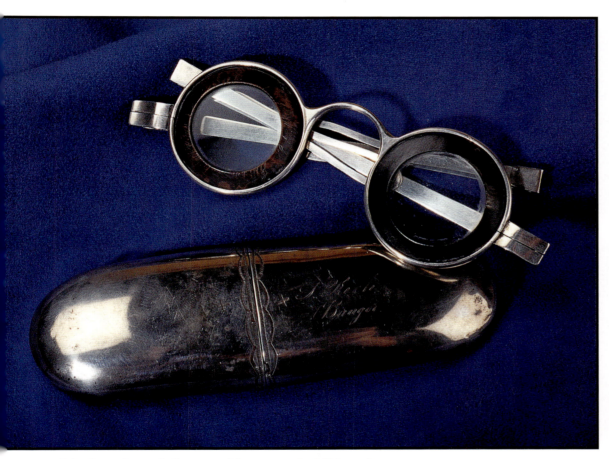

Pair of tortoise and silver round frames marked IS in a silver case engraved S. Rich, Bangor. Courtesy of John and Valda Tull.

Magnifiers

Specialized magnifying lenses for close hand work were also made in the 18th century, and two examples are shown. One is mounted above a spool of thread to magnify the eye of a needle. The other is mounted above tweezers. They both provide practical solutions for routine magnification.

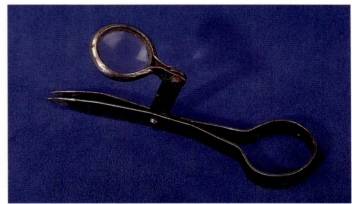

Above: Tweezers with attached magnifier. Courtesy of John and Valda Tull.

Left: Sewing aid with single lens mounted above a spool of black thread. Courtesy of John and Valda Tull.

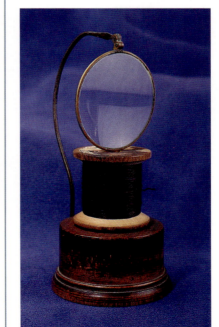

Bifocal lenses

Before the late 18th century, people who needed glasses for reading as well as for distance used two pair of glasses and switched back and forth. Cases for two eyeglasses from this period confirm the habit. Unhappy with this arrangement, American inventor Benjamin Franklin (1706-1790) took his two pair, cut the lenses horizontally, and made them into one pair which he could wear without interruption for both reading and distance viewing. The resulting invention of bifocal lenses by Franklin, about mid-century, is substantiated in a letter from Franklin to George Whatley, an optician in Philadelphia (ca. 1784): "...I had the glasses cut and half of each kind associated in the same circle. By this means, as I wear my spectacles constantly, I have only to move my eyes up or down, as I want to see distinctly far or near, the proper glasses being always ready." (Charles Letocha, "The Invention and Early Manufacture of Bifocals," *Survey of Ophthalmology*, Vol. 35, No. 3, Nov./Dec. 1990)

Methods of improving upon Franklin's invention have been undertaken up to the present for both bifocal and trifocal lenses. Using one or two pieces of glass for each lens, cut in different fashions, overlaid, or hinged, many variations have been produced.

John Richardson received an English patent (No. 2187) in 1797 for swinging side lenses and George Richards Elkington received an English patent in 1834 for a bifocal design. Elkington's improvement used wire to hold the upper lenses straight for distance viewing and the lower lenses at a 45º from the upper lenses for viewing near objects.

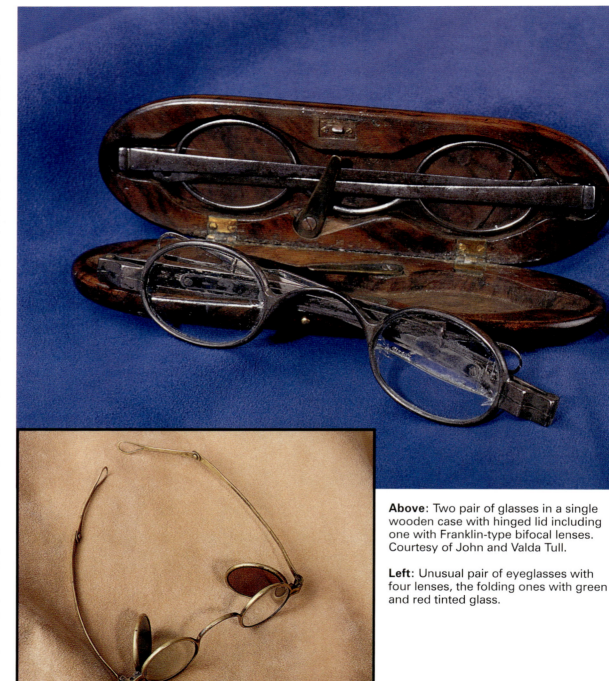

Above: Two pair of glasses in a single wooden case with hinged lid including one with Franklin-type bifocal lenses. Courtesy of John and Valda Tull.

Left: Unusual pair of eyeglasses with four lenses, the folding ones with green and red tinted glass.

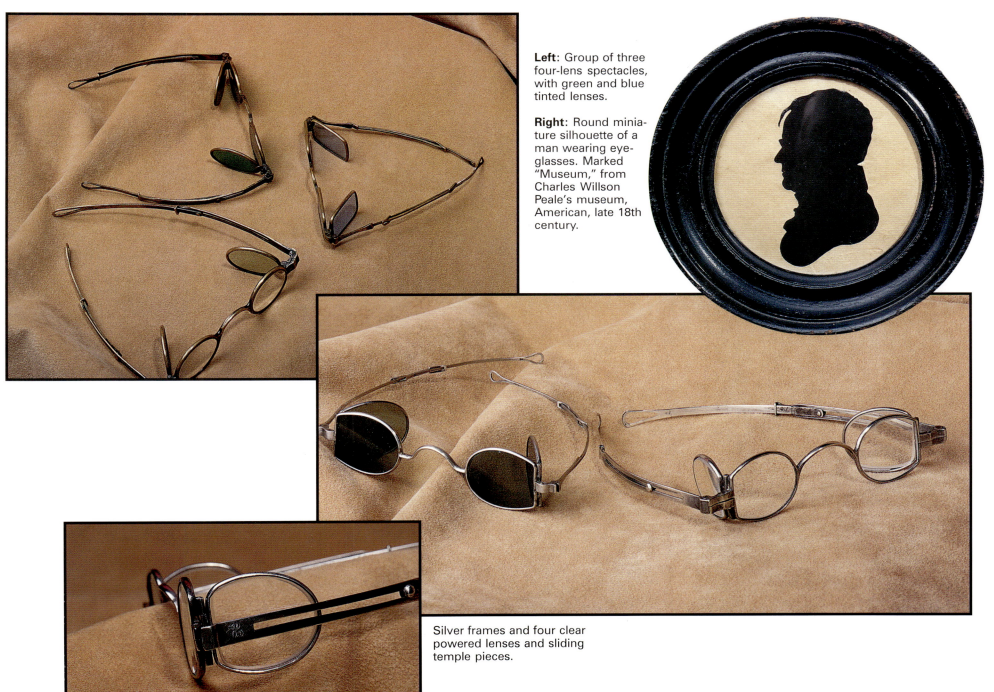

Left: Group of three four-lens spectacles, with green and blue tinted lenses.

Right: Round miniature silhouette of a man wearing eyeglasses. Marked "Museum," from Charles Willson Peale's museum, American, late 18th century.

Silver frames and four clear powered lenses and sliding temple pieces.

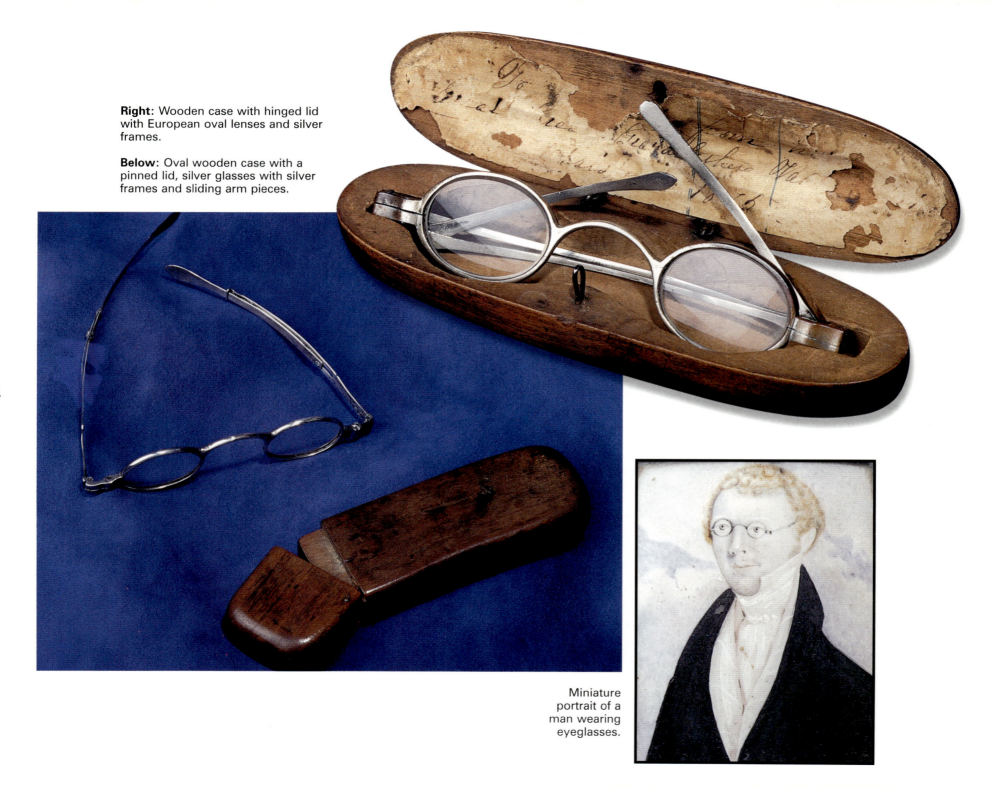

Right: Wooden case with hinged lid with European oval lenses and silver frames.

Below: Oval wooden case with a pinned lid, silver glasses with silver frames and sliding arm pieces.

Miniature portrait of a man wearing eyeglasses.

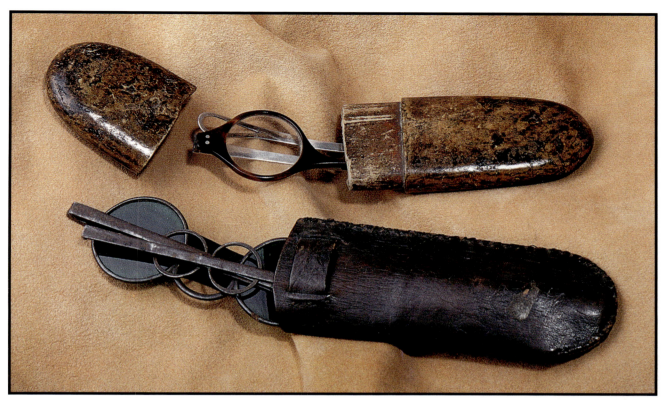

Left: Group of leather cases and tortoise with silver spectacles in hard oval two-part case, and green glass lenses in steel frames and soft leather case.

Below: Silver pair hallmarked by IH (possibly John Holmes, London, 1796) with black lacquer case.

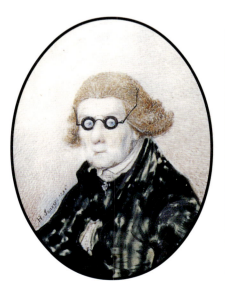
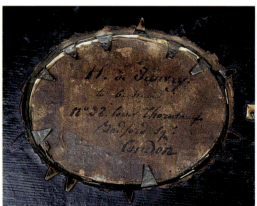

Miniature oval portrait of a man wearing eyeglasses, marked H. Janvey, 1796, and back inscribed "...Bedford Sq. London."

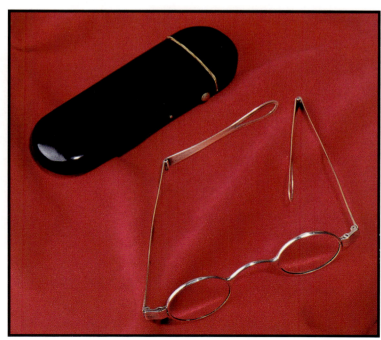

Scissors Glasses

Scissors glasses may have been developed in France after 1750, as early examples and illustrations seem to indicate, or in London, where optician George Adams patented scissors glasses in 1780. In scissors glasses, two round metal lens frames each were attached to a long stem and the stems were pinned with a rivet hinge at their ends. They were held under the nose for use. They became very popular in French society at the end of the eighteenth century, and therefore could also be found in England and America at that time. When they were made with an attached case at the end of their stems, they could also be considered as lorgnettes, which followed scissors glasses closely in design and popularity. Scissors-style glasses were made well into the 20th century.

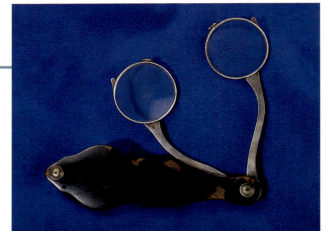

Scissors type folding lorgnette with tortoiseshell handle. Courtesy of John and Valda Tull.

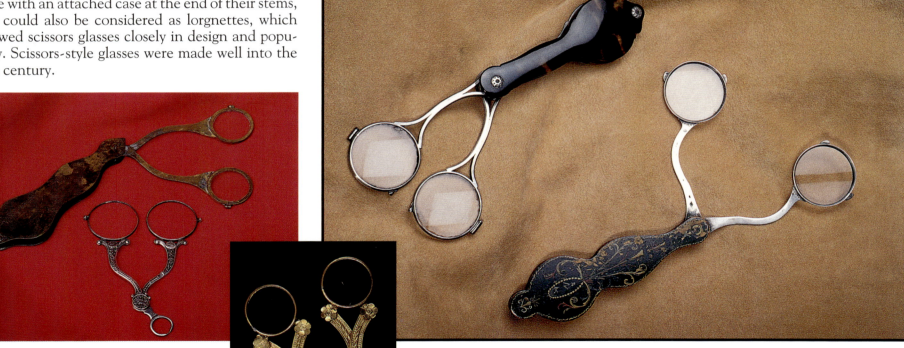

Two scissors-style eyepieces, 19th century, one brass German military officer's from Franco-Prussian War era, c. 1870. The other silver, possibly French, with European mark and 830.

Above: Two scissors type, one in decorated horn and the other in tortoiseshell.

Left: Scissors type lorgnette with gold tone metal cast handle. Courtesy of John and Valda Tull.

19TH CENTURY

The styles of eyeglasses dating from the early nineteenth century display the characteristics developed in the eighteenth century without dramatic change. Variations can be found in the sizes and shapes of the temple rings, and the arms may be straight, or adjustable: pivoting, folding, or sliding. The lenses are usually clear glass, but can be colored as well.

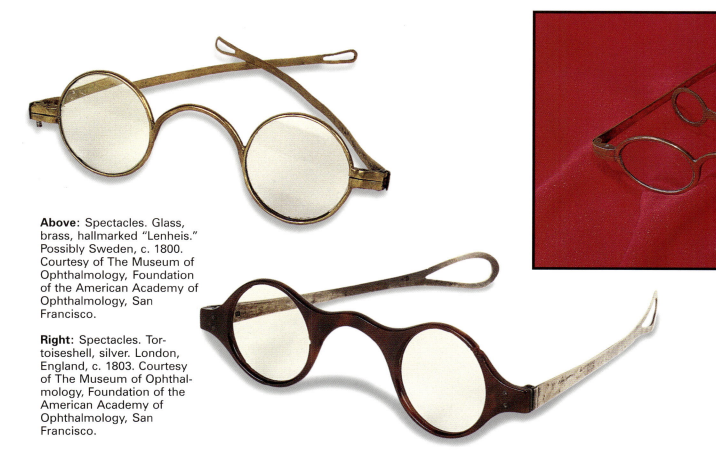

Above: Spectacles. Glass, brass, hallmarked "Lenheis." Possibly Sweden, c. 1800. Courtesy of The Museum of Ophthalmology, Foundation of the American Academy of Ophthalmology, San Francisco.

Right: Spectacles. Tortoiseshell, silver. London, England, c. 1803. Courtesy of The Museum of Ophthalmology, Foundation of the American Academy of Ophthalmology, San Francisco.

Brass eyeglasses with oval lenses and round end pieces, c. 1800.

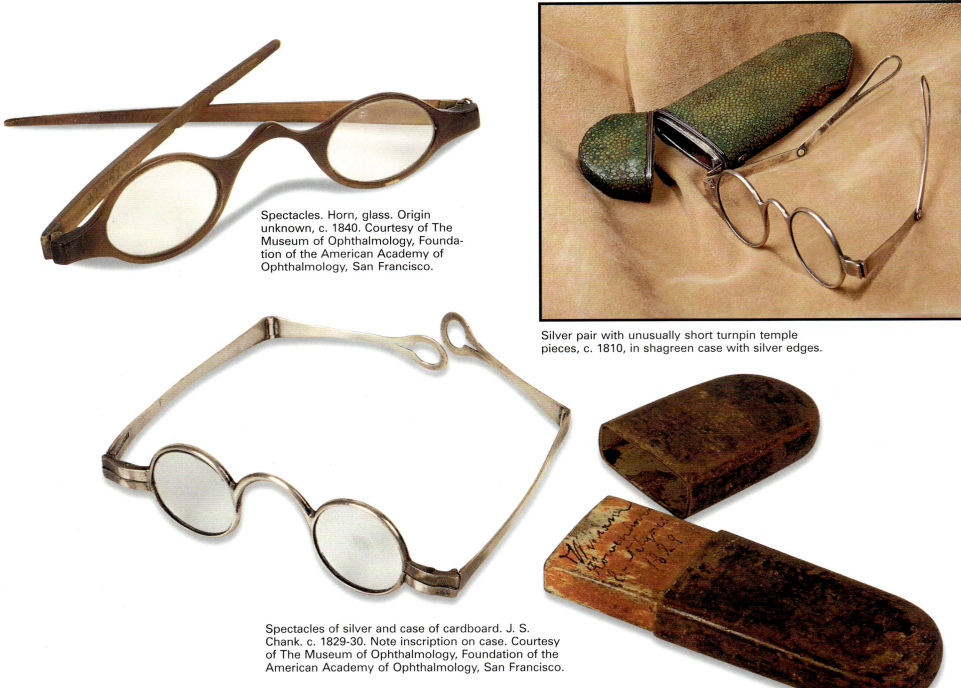

Spectacles. Horn, glass. Origin unknown, c. 1840. Courtesy of The Museum of Ophthalmology, Foundation of the American Academy of Ophthalmology, San Francisco.

Silver pair with unusually short turnpin temple pieces, c. 1810, in shagreen case with silver edges.

Spectacles of silver and case of cardboard. J. S. Chank. c. 1829-30. Note inscription on case. Courtesy of The Museum of Ophthalmology, Foundation of the American Academy of Ophthalmology, San Francisco.

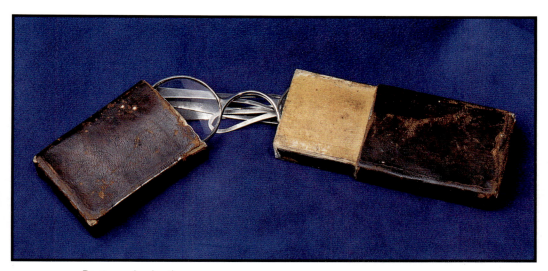

Rectangular leather case with silver spectacles.

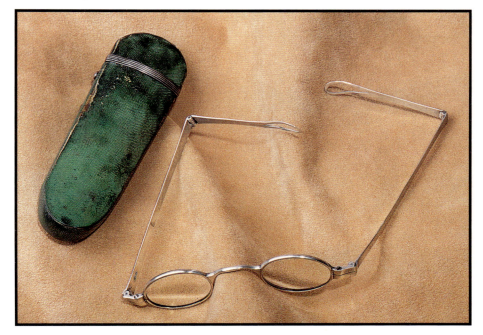

Green shagreen case, c. 1816, with oval lenses in silver frames.

Sliding Temples

In the early nineteenth century, temples frequently were made with sliding parts to extend them for dual use: from short for use under wigs to longer for use at the ears.

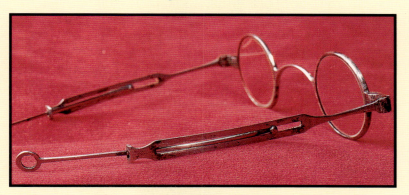

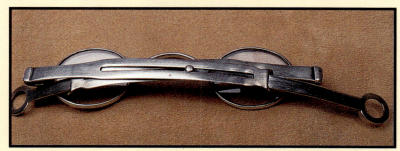

Details of the temple pieces of two silver frames with unusually small temple rings on the sliding arms.

Colored Lenses

Many colors of glass lenses were available for eyeglass lenses by 1800. They included smoke-gray, green, blue, and pink, each in many shades from dark to light. In 1832 in England, Elias Solomons patented lenses made from amber. Many people studied and produced lenses of various colors and most were promoted as being better than clear for various reasons. The claims ranged from soothing and cooler in the early nineteenth century to absorbing dangerous ultraviolet and infrared rays in the early twentieth century.

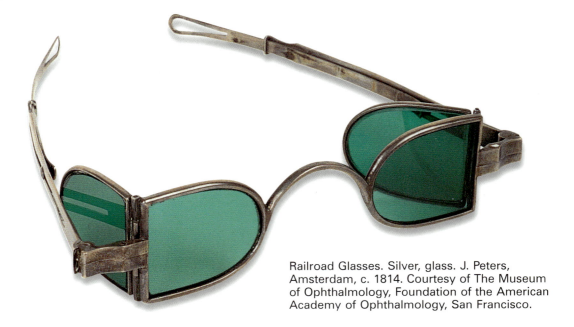

Railroad Glasses. Silver, glass. J. Peters, Amsterdam, c. 1814. Courtesy of The Museum of Ophthalmology, Foundation of the American Academy of Ophthalmology, San Francisco.

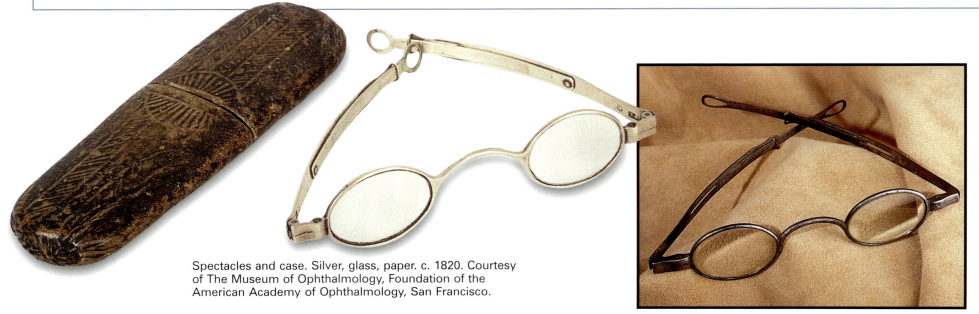

Spectacles and case. Silver, glass, paper. c. 1820. Courtesy of The Museum of Ophthalmology, Foundation of the American Academy of Ophthalmology, San Francisco.

Steel-framed eyewear with sliding side pieces and small oval lenses, c. 1820. Courtesy of Barbara Blau.

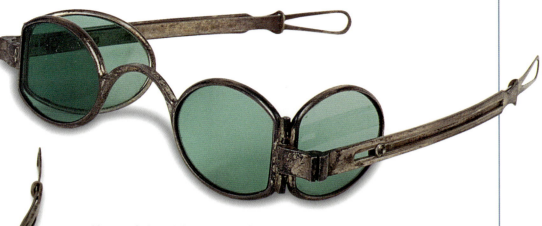

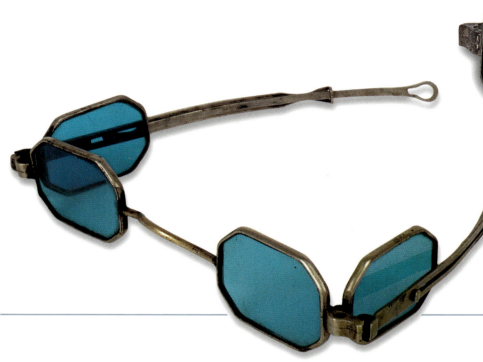

Above: Colored Spectacles. Silver. E. Hughes, c. 1840. Courtesy of The Museum of Ophthalmology, Foundation of the American Academy of Ophthalmology, San Francisco.

Left: Colored glass spectacles, steel and glass. c. 1825. Courtesy of The Museum of Ophthalmology, Foundation of the American Academy of Ophthalmology, San Francisco.

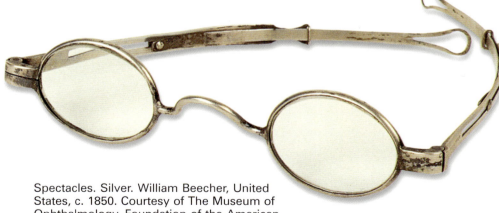

Spectacles. Silver. William Beecher, United States, c. 1850. Courtesy of The Museum of Ophthalmology, Foundation of the American Academy of Ophthalmology, San Francisco.

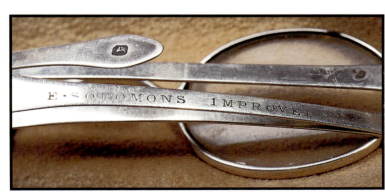

Detail of the English hallmark and inscription "E. Solomons Improved" on silver frames.

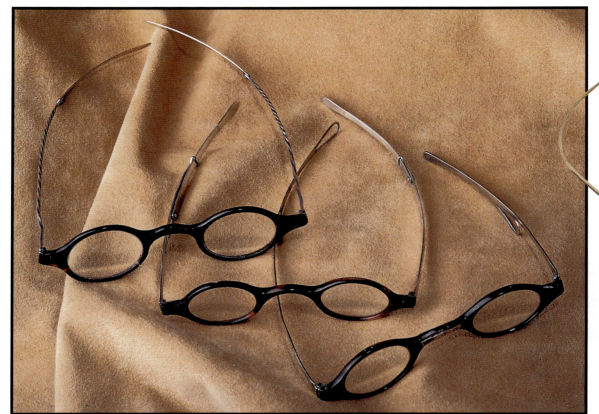

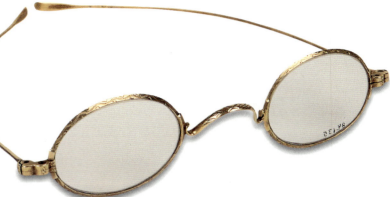

Above: Spectacles. Gold. United States, c. 1850. Courtesy of The Museum of Ophthalmology, Foundation of the American Academy of Ophthalmology, San Francisco.

Left: Tortoiseshell frames with nose piece repaired with silver, and silver ear pieces. Tortoiseshell frames with twisted silver arms. Tortoise frames with sliding silver arms.

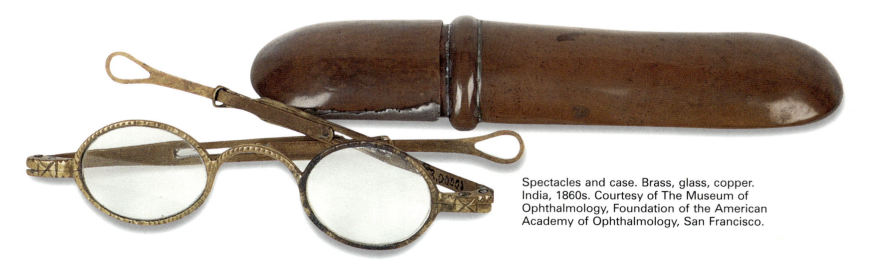

Spectacles and case. Brass, glass, copper. India, 1860s. Courtesy of The Museum of Ophthalmology, Foundation of the American Academy of Ophthalmology, San Francisco.

Specialized Lenses

In the early nineteenth century, opticians experimented with ways to improve lenses as their profession gained scientific accuracy as well as widespread acceptance. As more people were using eyeglasses, their vision problems were constantly being studied and became better understood. Hand-ground lenses of c. 1820 can be seen easily on the biconvex example shown which were made in gold frames by the McAllister firm of Philadelphia.

In 1836, German immigrant lens maker Isaac Schnaitman of Philadelphia received a patent for a new design for bifocal lenses. His design had two focal centers ground into the single lens.

An unusual eyeglass design is shown with prism lenses cut at a sharp angle so the wearer can read while lying down in bed. The style remains rare because it probably did not sell well.

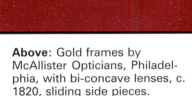

Above: Gold frames by McAllister Opticians, Philadelphia, with bi-concave lenses, c. 1820, sliding side pieces.

Below: Bifocal glasses by Isaac Schnaitman where the upper part of the lens is for distance. Courtesy of John and Valda Tull.

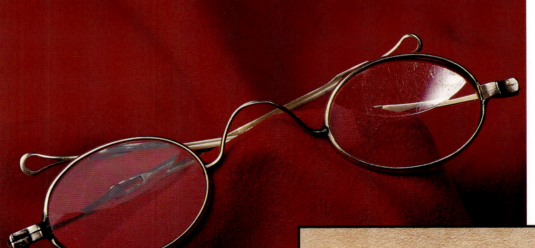

Left: Gold rimmed, bi-focal glasses patented in 1836 by Isaac Schnaitman of Philadelphia, with sliding temple pieces.

Below: Prism glasses for reading while lying back, as for reading in bed.

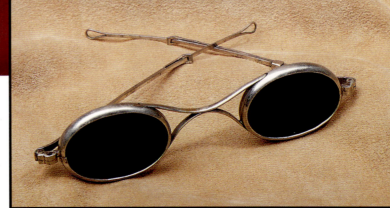

Inscribed Numbers

Sometimes inscribed numbers are found on the temples of eyeglasses, especially those made c. 1850, usually near the hinges. In England and America they represent inches, but in France they represented pounces (13 inches = 12 pounces). When these numbers are below 40, they usually represent the focal powers of the lenses, such those intended for viewing text 12, 16, or 20 inches (or pounces) from the eyes.

When numbers inscribed on the temples exceed 40, they may represent the approximate age of the intended wearer, such as age 50 or 60. (In the twentieth century, eyeglasses could be ordered by the wearer's age group from the Sears and Roebuck Company's mail order catalogs from 1961 to 1964 [see examples in the section on the twentieth century].)

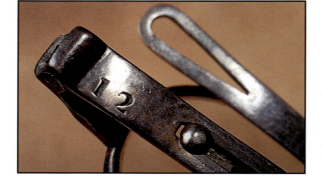
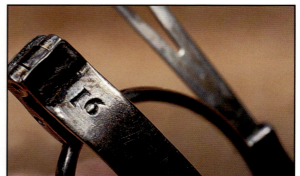

These pictures show different numbers on the frames: numbers 36 and below indicate focal length, while numbers 40 and above indicate the approximate age of the wearer.

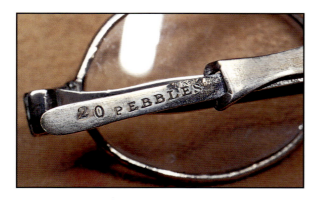
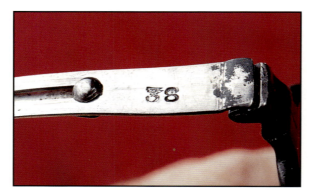
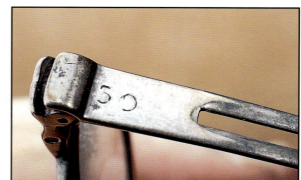

Three hand-held magnifiers: one with bone handle and thick brass frame. One with open silver hinged handle and frame, and one with mother of pearl hinged handle and silver frame in a leather case. Courtesy of John and Valda Tull.

Magnifiers

Hand-held single magnifying glasses were quite fashionable and popular throughout the nineteenth century and can be found in numerous materials and styles, including folding ones. They are sometimes jeweled and their cases can be of plain or fine materials with little or elaborate ornamentation.

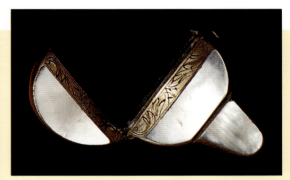

Left: Mother of pearl and brass case for a magnifier. Courtesy of John and Valda Tull.

Below: Jewelry pendants with magnifiers and jeweled covers, costume jewelry, mid-20th century. Courtesy of John and Valda Tull.

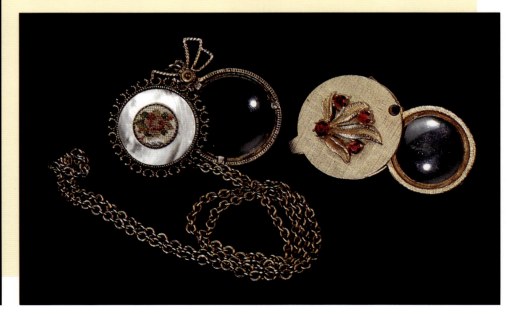

Monocles

Single lenses also were mounted for wearing on one eye, and these we call monocles today. They were frameless or framed with gold, silver, tortoiseshell, and horn. J. W. Rosenthal writes that early "monocles were certainly used for corrective purposes, later ones were often worn purely as a matter of fashion in imitation of the aristocracy." (*Spectacles and Other Vision Aids*, p. 230) The fashion for wearing monocles in Europe developed in the late 18th century when it was considered elegant to peer through a lens with an arrogant air. The fashion subsided, reappeared about 1820, and reappeared again at the end of the nineteenth century. The single round lens was held by the upper and lower eyelids alone. The monocle was usually attached to a string, ribbon, or chain which could be worn loosely around the neck or attached to a vest pocket, hairpin, or button to prevent the monocle from falling to the floor. When used for better vision, monocles could be ground for reading or distance vision. When used for dramatic affect, it was an unground glass.

Monoculars

Monoculars are single-eye telescopes with sliding tubes, and they were popularly used to spy on other patrons in a theater. They are differentiated from *binoculars* (called "opera glasses" at the theater and "field glasses" for horse races) which are two monoculars joined together. Monoculars have two lenses, held parallel one in front of the other, that can be moved for magnification to an appropriate focal distance. They remained popular throughout the nineteenth century and can be found alone as well as mounted on walking sticks, perfume bottles, and other fashion accessories.

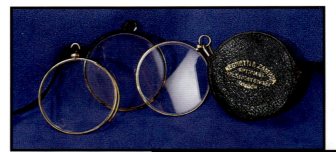

Three monocles: one in gold frame on black ribbon with leather case marked Negretti & Zambra Opticians, 122 Regent Street, London, mid-19th century; one on black string with metal keepers on the frame to support the lens at your eye, mid-19th century; and a monocle with plastic tortoise frame, mid-20th century. Courtesy of John and Valda Tull.

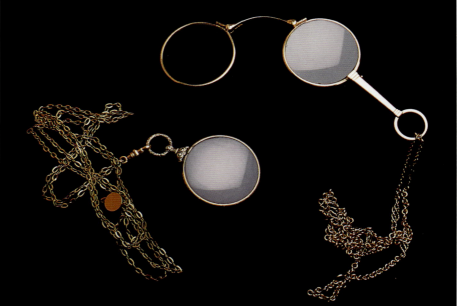

Right: Monocle with gold frame and gold chain. Lorgnette in gold frame with handle, ring end, and gold chain. Courtesy of Barbara Blau.

Below: Two telescoping monocular opera glasses, one of ivory with gold rings and one of brass with turquoise stones, late 19th century. Courtesy of John and Valda Tull.

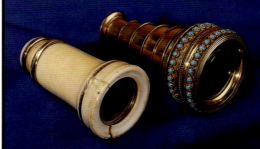

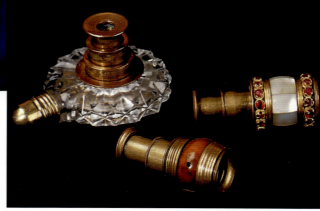

Group of monocular opera glasses, one fashioned as a perfume bottle and two as charms, late 19th century. Courtesy of John and Valda Tull.

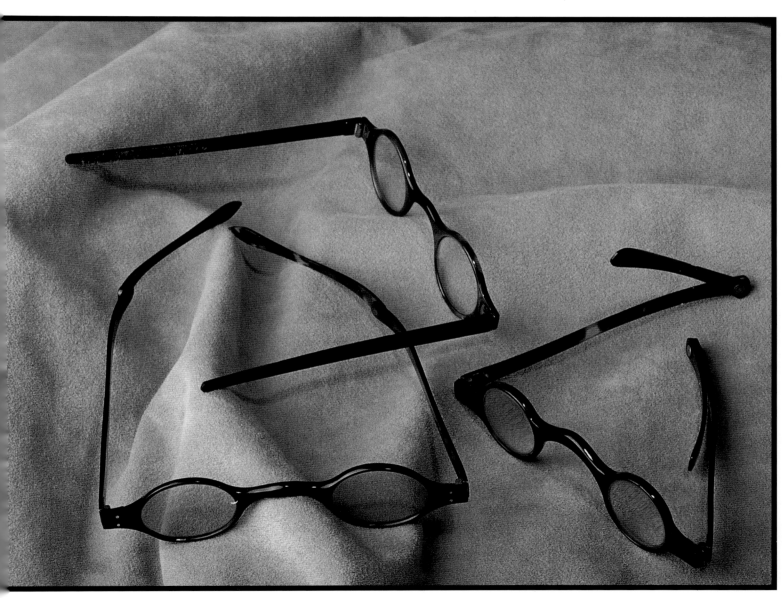

Three tortoiseshell frames, mid-19th century, with various arm styles, but none that slide.

Tortoiseshell and Horn Frames

Eyeglass frames and cases have been made with cow horn and tortoiseshell for centuries. The shell of hawksbill sea turtles grows in rigid plates that can be fused and molded when heated. This material then can be cut to any shape. Hand-made tortoiseshell eyeglass parts were known in the eighteenth century, and it became fashionable to have frames entirely made of tortoiseshell in the mid-to-late nineteenth century. Many styles can be found. Likewise, horn (colored lighter than most tortoiseshell) became popular as an eyeglass frame material in the late nineteenth century. The temples on these tortoise frames were usually long and straight and the lenses were usually round, until c. 1930.

Cases for eyeglasses were made from tortoiseshell from the eighteenth century. In the nineteenth century, they became decorated with fancy inlays of mother of pearl and engraved silver plaques.

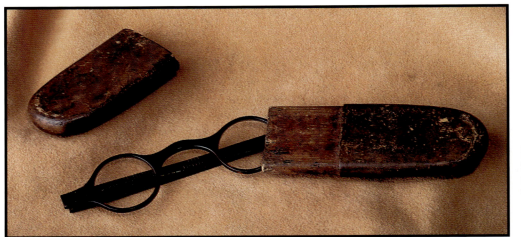

Pair of tortoiseshell frames with oval lenses and oval leather case with sliding end.

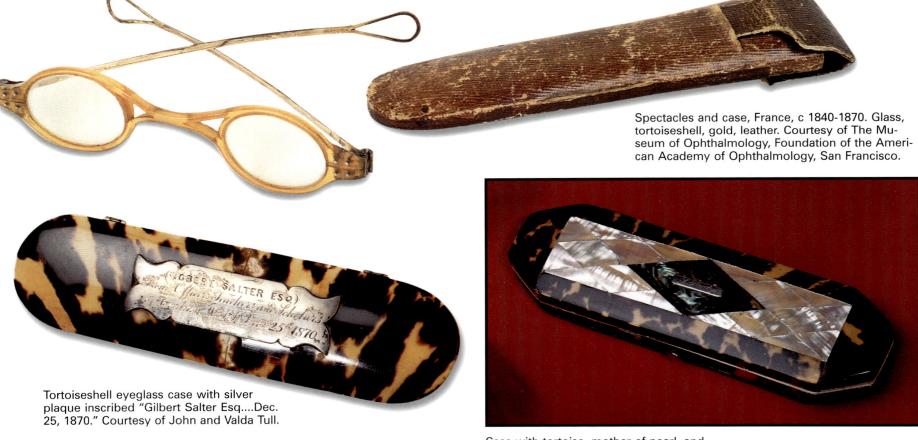

Spectacles and case, France, c 1840-1870. Glass, tortoiseshell, gold, leather. Courtesy of The Museum of Ophthalmology, Foundation of the American Academy of Ophthalmology, San Francisco.

Tortoiseshell eyeglass case with silver plaque inscribed "Gilbert Salter Esq....Dec. 25, 1870." Courtesy of John and Valda Tull.

Case with tortoise, mother of pearl, and shell with silver engraved S. Plenty.

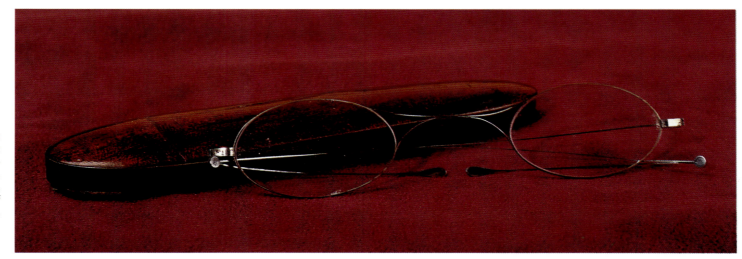

Silver wire rim spectacles with folding arms, K-shaped wire bridge, and wooden case, c. 1880. Courtesy of John and Valda Tull.

Wire Frames

The industrial revolution brought efficient change to every industry, including that of eyeglasses. By the middle of the nineteenth century, wire could be drawn mechanically to provide strong steel and gold for eyeglass frames. Around 1875 wire temples were made with curving ear pieces that wrapped behind the ears. Wire cables were made later, and by c.1900 cable temples were available and stronger than wire.

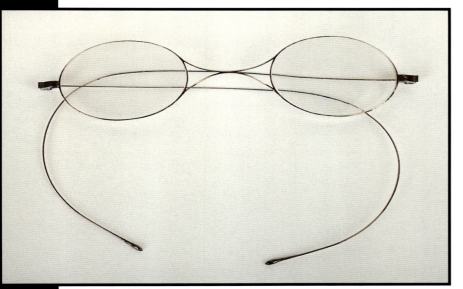

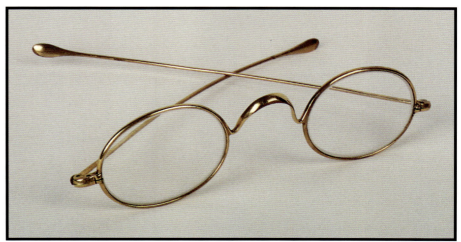

Above: Spectacles. Glass, fine steel wire with x-bridge, c. 1870. Courtesy of The Museum of Ophthalmology, Foundation of the American Academy of Ophthalmology, San Francisco.

Right: Spectacles. Gold, glass. c. 1890-1900. Courtesy of The Museum of Ophthalmology, Foundation of the American Academy of Ophthalmology, San Francisco.

MCALLISTER OPTICIANS

The McAllister family of opticians served their communities for many generations in Philadelphia, Pennsylvania, and elsewhere, from 1799 to 1971. A surprising variety of eyeglasses and cases bearing their marks and labels has been preserved today, making the study of one family's work particularly intriguing.

The following chart has been compiled to aid the dating and identity of McAllister made and/or sold eyeglasses and cases.

Name	Working Dates	Address
In Philadelphia, Pennsylvania:		
John McAllister, Sr.	c.1799-1812	48 Chestnut St.
McAllister & Son	c.1812-1830	48 Chestnut St.
John McAllister, Jr. & Co.	c. 1830-1836	48 Chestnut St.
McAllister & Co. Opticians	c.1836-1854	1407 Chestnut St.
McAllister & Brother	c.1854-1865	728 Chestnut St.
William Y. McAllister	c.1865-1881	728 Chestnut St.
McAllister Optician	c.1881-1882	1226 Chestnut St.
J. Cook McAllister	c.1882-1928	1721 1/2 Chestnut St.
"	"	No. 9 South 16th St.
William Mitchell McAllister	c.1882-1905	720 Chestnut St.
McAllister Opt. Co. Ltd.	?-?	705 Chestnut St.
McAllister Opt. Co.	?-?	1113 or 1116 Chestnut St.
In New York City, New York:		
Thomas H. McAllister	c.1863-1900	49 Nassau Street
In Baltimore, Maryland:		
Francis W. McAllister	c.1878-1920	113 or 118 North Charles St.
Francis W. Mc Allister	?-?	3 North Charles St.
John W. McAllister	c. 1920-1971	

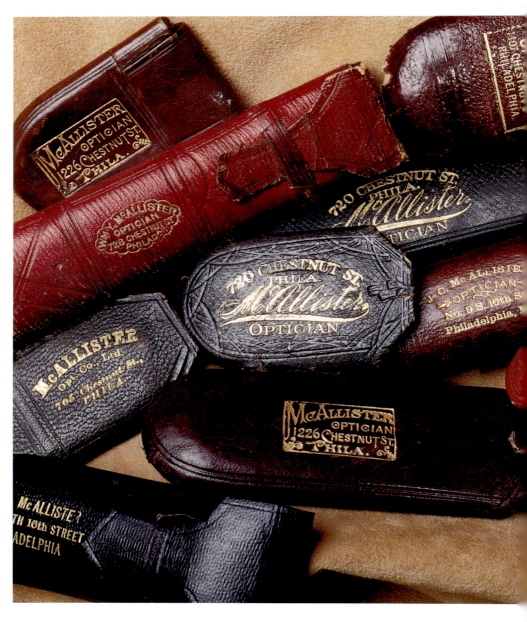

Eyeglass cases all marked McAllister and dating from over a hundred-year period.

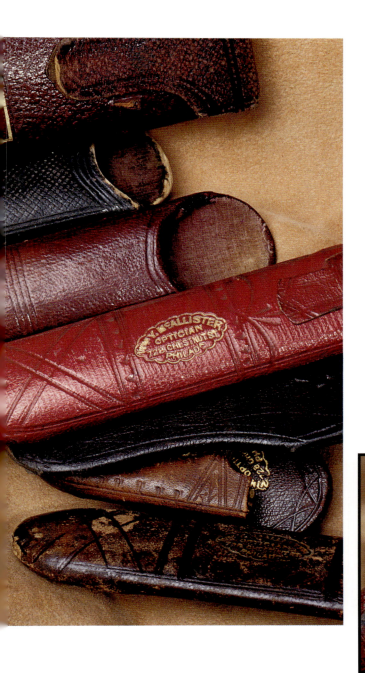

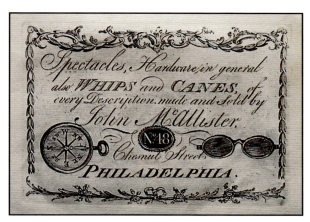

Engraved paper of John McAllister 48 Chestnut Street.

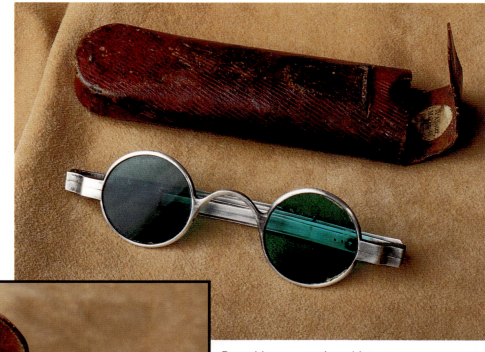

Round lenses continued into the nineteenth century; green lenses are an example of this. Red leather case with McAllister paper label.

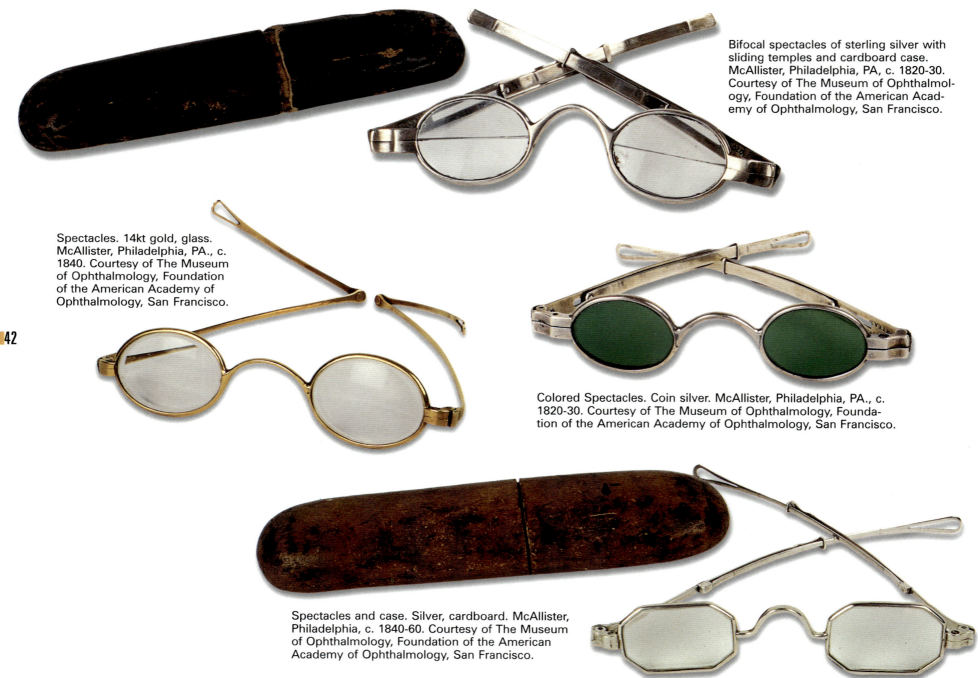

Bifocal spectacles of sterling silver with sliding temples and cardboard case. McAllister, Philadelphia, PA, c. 1820-30. Courtesy of The Museum of Ophthalmology, Foundation of the American Academy of Ophthalmology, San Francisco.

Spectacles. 14kt gold, glass. McAllister, Philadelphia, PA., c. 1840. Courtesy of The Museum of Ophthalmology, Foundation of the American Academy of Ophthalmology, San Francisco.

Colored Spectacles. Coin silver. McAllister, Philadelphia, PA., c. 1820-30. Courtesy of The Museum of Ophthalmology, Foundation of the American Academy of Ophthalmology, San Francisco.

Spectacles and case. Silver, cardboard. McAllister, Philadelphia, c. 1840-60. Courtesy of The Museum of Ophthalmology, Foundation of the American Academy of Ophthalmology, San Francisco.

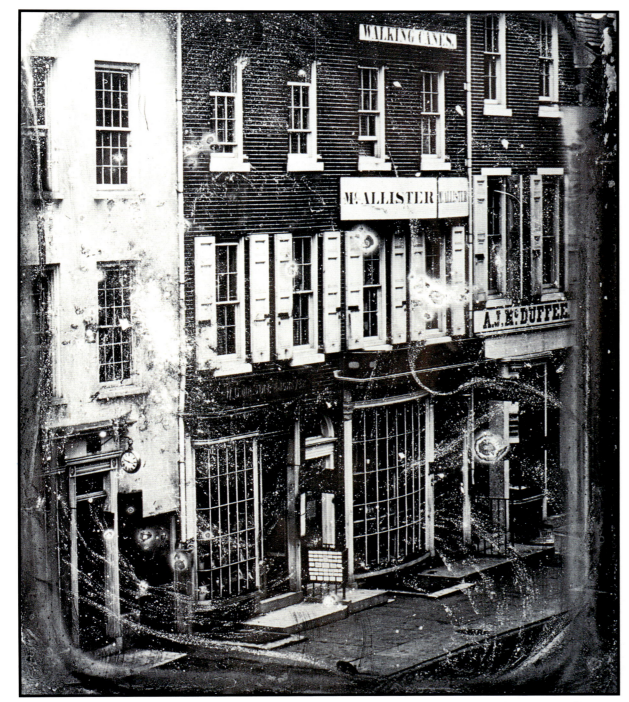

Photograph of the McAllister optical shop of 1843 at 48 Chestnut Street in Philadelphia. Courtesy of John and Valda Tull.

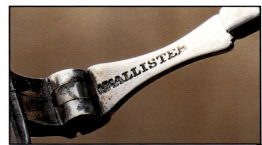

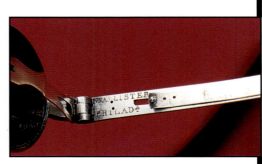

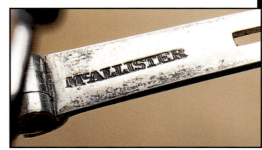

Other McAllister marks on silver frames.

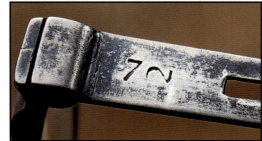

Silver McAllister pair with nearsighted lenses and indication for it as 7/2.

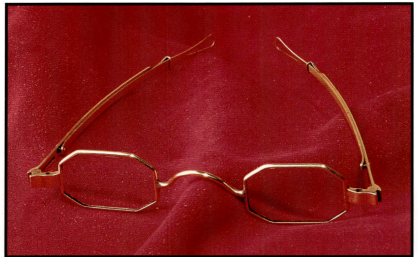

Gold McAllister glasses with octagonal lenses, c. 1840-50, marked McAllister.

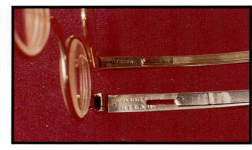

Gold McAllister frames showing two different marks.

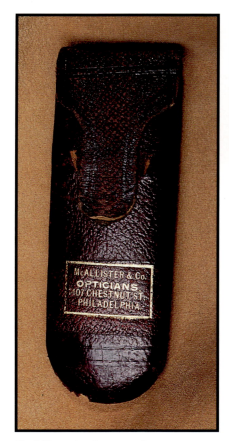

McAllister leather eyeglass case, c. 1840-50, from 1407 Chestnut Street in Philadelphia.

Spectacles. Silver, glass. McAllister, Philadelphia, c. 1850. Courtesy of The Museum of Ophthalmology, Foundation of the American Academy of Ophthalmology, San Francisco.

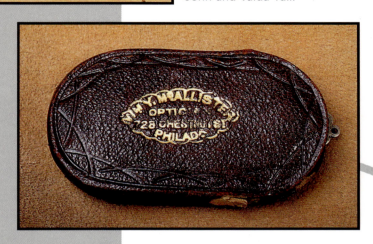

Label, Sold by McAllister & Brother, 728 Chestnut Street, Philadelphia, c. 1856-65. Courtesy of John and Valda Tull.

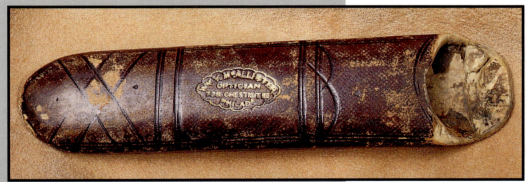

McAllister leather eyeglass cases prior to 1882, of different shapes, and with different street numbers on Chestnut Street in Philadelphia.

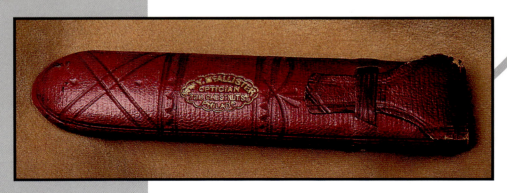

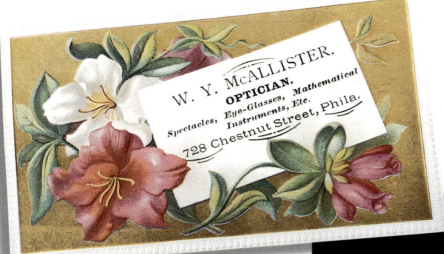

Trade card of W. Y. McAllister at 728 Chestnut Street, Philadelphia.

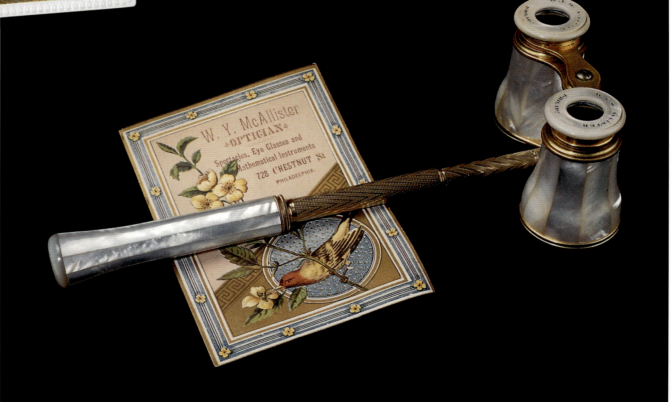

Opera glasses and trade card both marked W.Y. McAllister. Courtesy of John and Valda Tull.

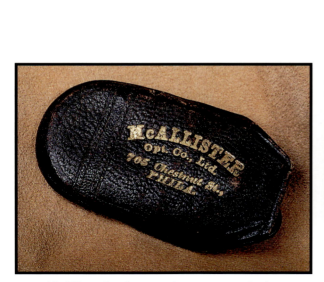

McAllister leather eyeglass case marked McAllister Opt. Co. Ltd., 705 Chestnut St.

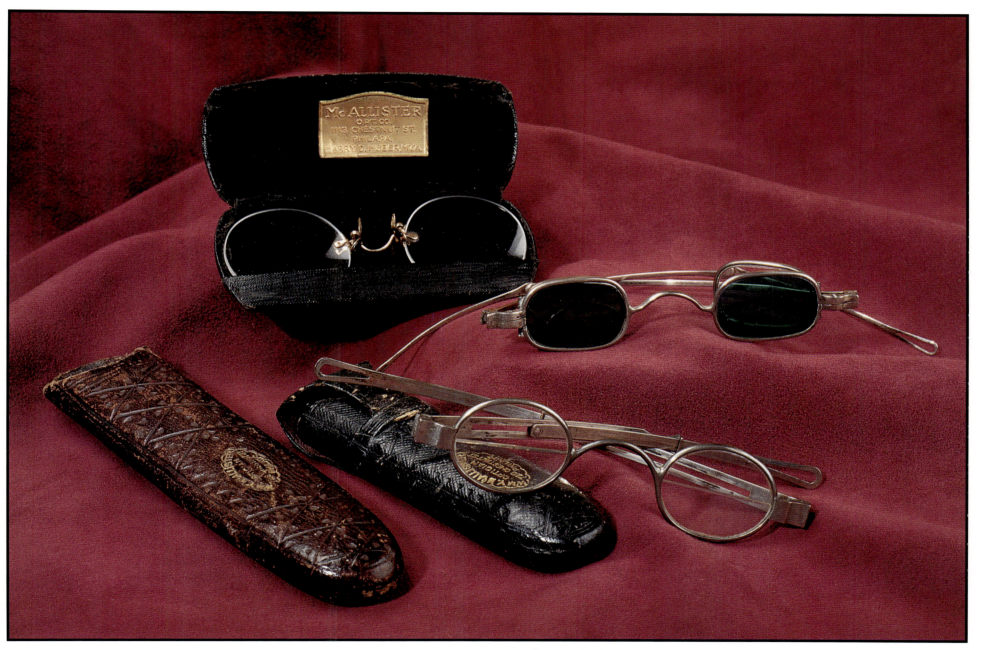

Three pair of McAllister Opt. Co. glasses and cases, gold label reads "Harry D. Huber". Courtesy of John and Valda Tull.

CASES

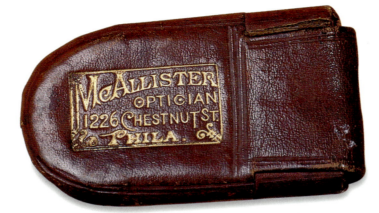
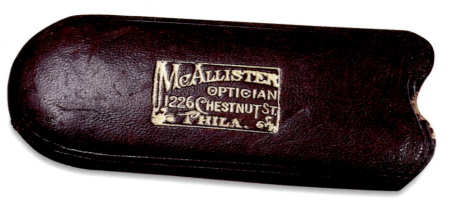
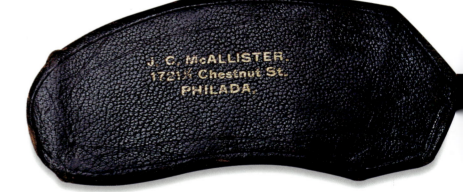
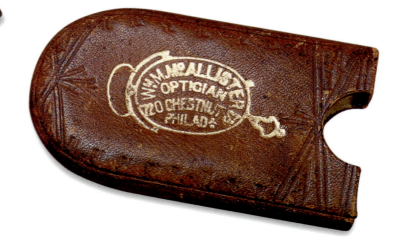
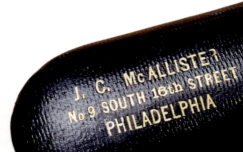

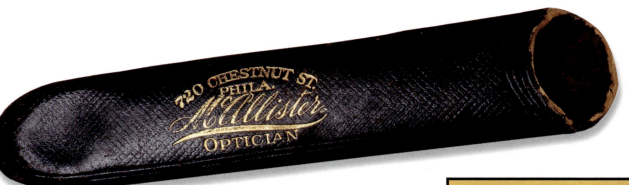
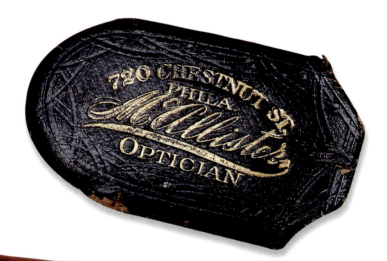
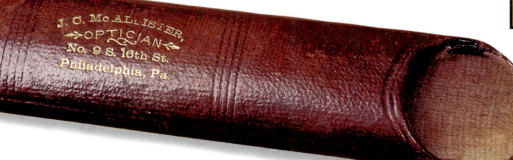
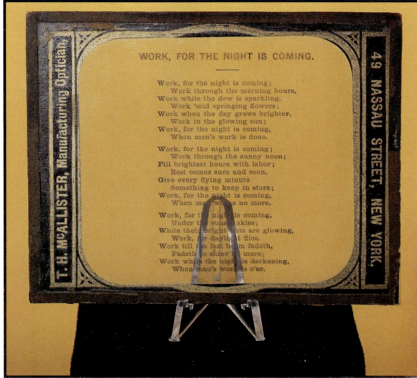

Projector slide marked T.H. McAllister, Manufacturing Optician, 49 Nassau Street, and poem "Work, For the Night is coming." Courtesy of John and Valda Tull.

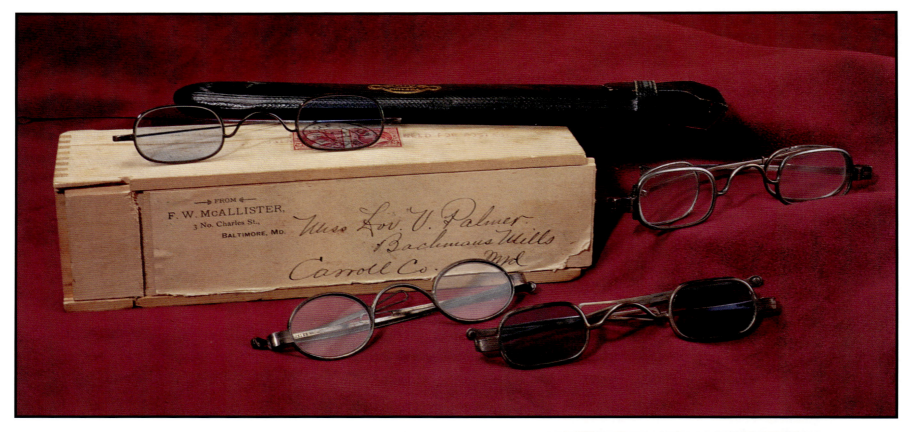

Above: Group of McAllister items covering a wide time period, including eyeglasses, cases, shipping boxes, projector slide, stereo picture, and advertising cards. One with the mailing box, long temples and unique long case. Courtesy of John and Valda Tull

Right: Eyeglasses, c. 1820-30, are much older than the case. Black case patented Nov.1907, marked F.W. McAllister 113 N. Charles St. Baltimore, Maryland. (Frank McAllister 1853-1920) with a stereoscope printed card. Courtesy of John and Valda Tull

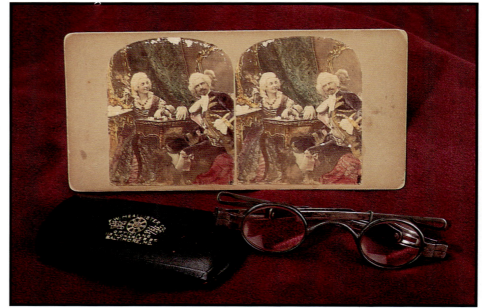

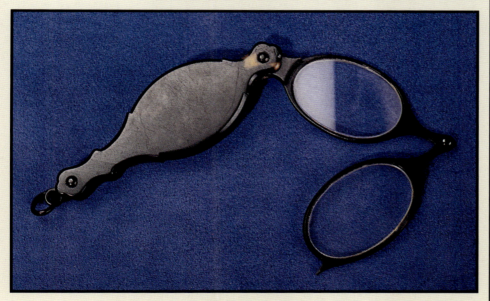

Top: French style tortoiseshell folding lorgnette with short pierced handle, c. 1840-1900. Courtesy of John and Valda Tull.

Center: Folding black tortoiseshell lorgnette. Courtesy of John and Valda Tull.

Bottom: Lorgnette with white shell case and steel rims.

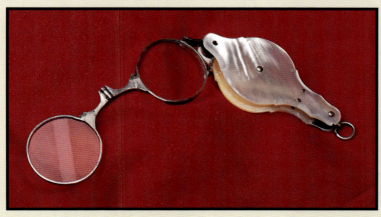

LORGNETTES

Lornettes are double lens eyeglasses made for women that are attached to a handle, and sometimes the handle is hinged to fold and become the case. There are no temple pieces on lorgnettes or pince-nez eyeglasses. Their design seems to have closely followed that of scissors glasses, which were popular at the end of the eighteenth century (see section on scissors glasses).

English optician George Adams designed a case for eyeglasses in 1785 so they could be carried conveniently in a pocket. In this design, oval metal eyeglass frames were pivot-hinged to a case comprised of two flat and shaped sides, usually made from tortoiseshell, metal, or other stiff materials.

The sides often conformed in shape to the eyeglass frame. The frames could be straight at the bridge or folded to swing into the case. This is one style of lorgnette.

An English patent (No. 3031) was issued in 1889 to George Bussey for "improvements in the application of eyeglasses and spectacles to the handles of umbrellas, walking sticks,... parasols,... whips, fans, and other articles of like nature, by pivoting the same in slots or recesses formed therein." An improved closing arrangement in the handle of lorgnette glasses was patented (No. 15065) in England in 1895 by Jean Fehl, a goldsmith in Hanau, Germany.

Lorgnette hand-held eyeglasses also were made throughout the nineteenth century without attached cases, and many designs remain. Robert Bretell Bate received an English patent (No. 5124) in 1825 for a spring-loaded design to unfold lorgnettes easily and quickly. Toward the end of the nineteenth century, lorgnettes with extremely long handles became popular. One shown has a long ear trumpet handle to help its wearer both see and hear better.

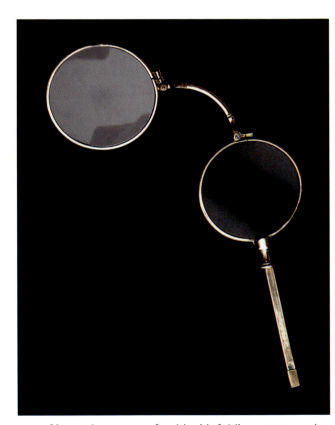

Above: Lorgnette of gold with folding center and square handle with repaired end (incomplete, rings missing). Courtesy of Mary Ann Berlangieri. $250

Right: Gold frame folding eyeglasses on long handle. Folding tortoiseshell eyeglasses with short ring handle. Folding gold rim eyeglasses on short loop handle. Oliver Goldsmith Eyewear Ltd.

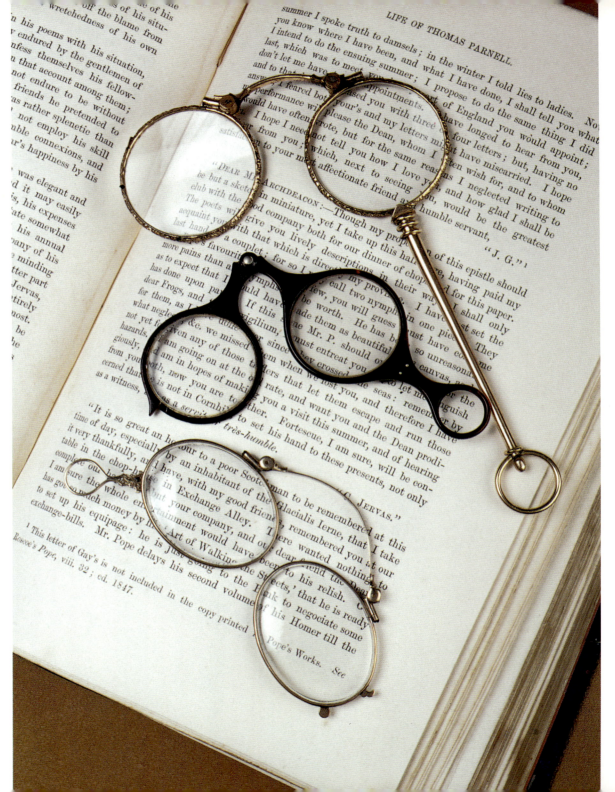

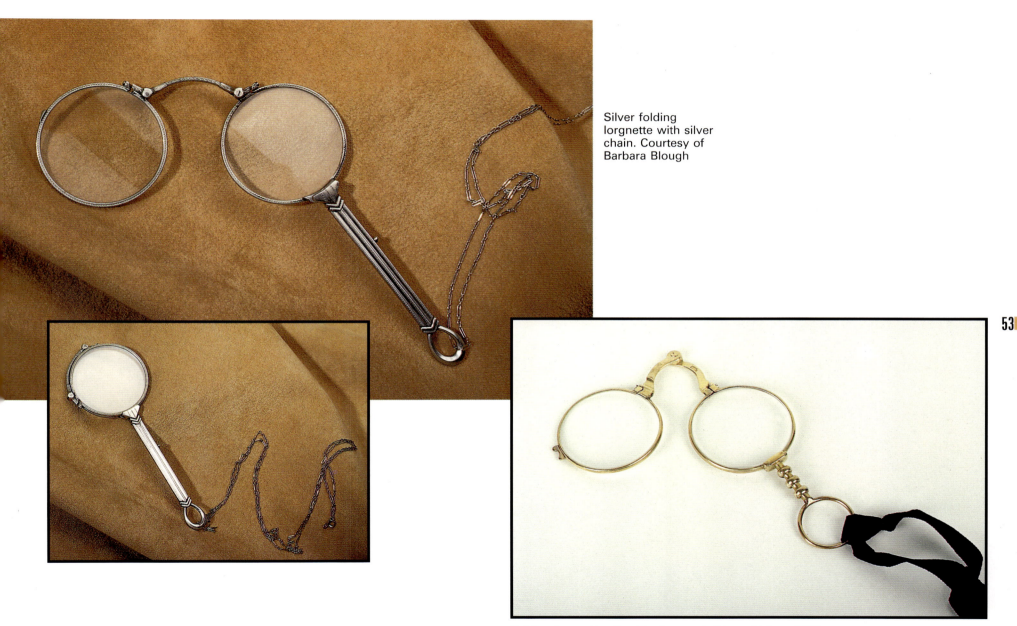

Silver folding lorgnette with silver chain. Courtesy of Barbara Blough

Folding lorgnette of gold, glass and ribbon, Irish, c. 1870. Courtesy of The Musuem of Ophthalmology, Foundation of the American Academy of Ophthalmology, San Francisco

Below & right: Lorgnette of plated gold and glass, c. 1880. Courtesy of The Musuem of Ophthalmology, Foundation of the American Academy of Ophthalmology, San Francisco

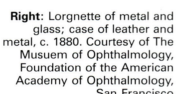

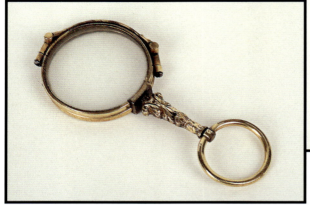

Right: Lorgnette of metal and glass; case of leather and metal, c. 1880. Courtesy of The Musuem of Ophthalmology, Foundation of the American Academy of Ophthalmology, San Francisco

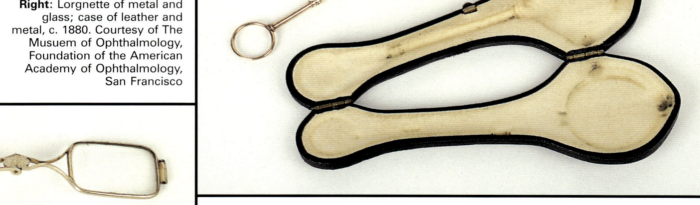

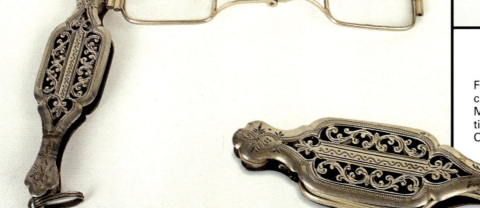

Folding lorgnette. Metal and glass. c.1880-1900. Courtesy of The Museum of Ophthalmology, Foundation of the American Academy of Ophthalmology, San Francisco.

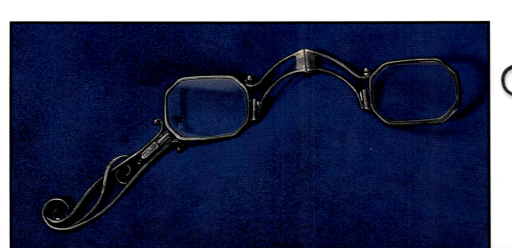

Left: Folding lorgnette. Silver. Origin unknown. c. 1895. Courtesy of The Museum of Ophthalmology, Foundation of the American Academy of Ophthalmology, San Francisco.

Below: Lorgnette. Gold-plated, sterling silver, glass. Cattail motif on handle. c. 1880-1910. Courtesy of The Museum of Ophthalmology, Foundation of the American Academy of Ophthalmology, San Francisco.

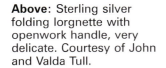

Above: Sterling silver folding lorgnette with openwork handle, very delicate. Courtesy of John and Valda Tull.

Right: Folding lorgnette with openwork gilded silver handle. Courtesy of John and Valda Tull

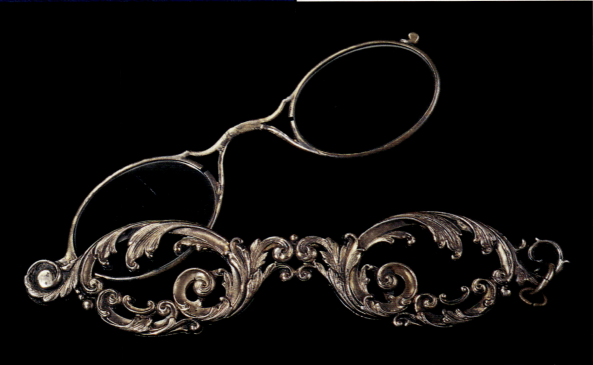

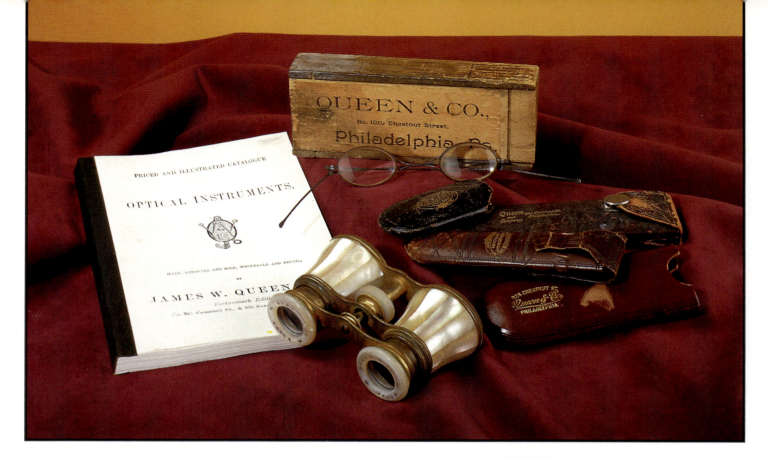

Above: Group of associated items from James W. Queen & Co. 924 Chestnut St. & 925 Sansom St., Philadelphia, including a reprint of the 1879 catalog of optical instruments. Courtesy of John and Valda Tull.

Right: Opera glasses with white porcelain handle and case with pink roses, brass and mother-of-pearl eyepieces. Courtesy of John and Valda Tull.

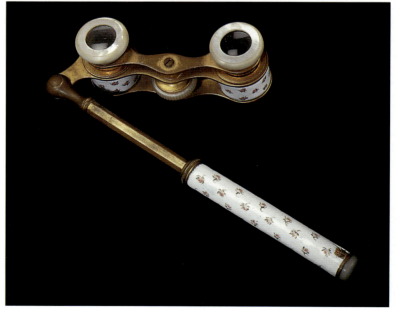

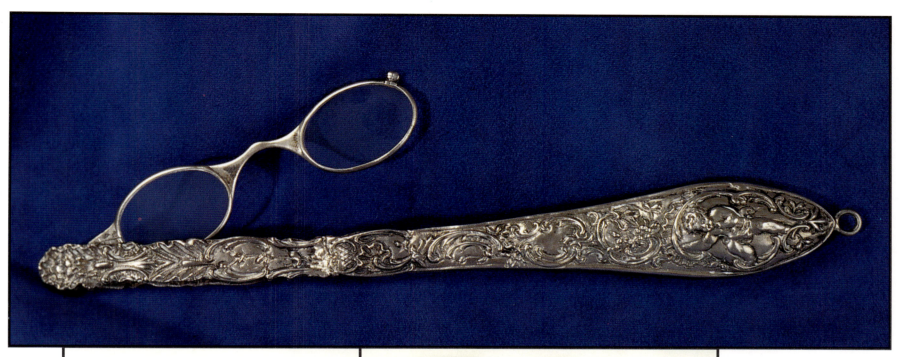

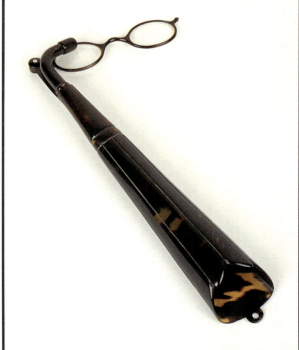
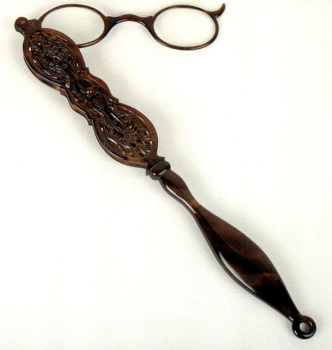

Above: European silver lorgnette with long repoussé handle including cupid. Courtesy of John and Valda Tull.

Lower left: Folding lorgnette. Tortoiseshell, metal. Handle is also an ear trumpet. Origin unknown, c. 1880. Courtesy of The Museum of Ophthalmology, Foundation of the American Academy of Ophthalmology, San Francisco.

Lower right: Folding lorgnette. Tortoiseshell and glass. c. 1880. Courtesy of The Museum of Ophthalmology, Foundation of the American Academy of Ophthalmology, San Francisco.

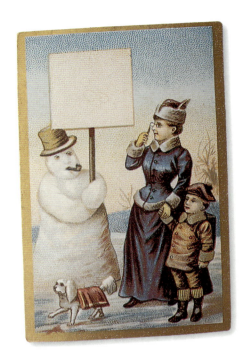

Above: Printed paper postcard depicting a snowman, woman with lorgnette, and child. Courtesy of John and Valda Tull

Right: Folding lorgnette. Tortoiseshell, glass, and gold. c. 1890. Courtesy of The Museum of Ophthalmology, Foundation of the American Academy of Ophthalmology, San Francisco.

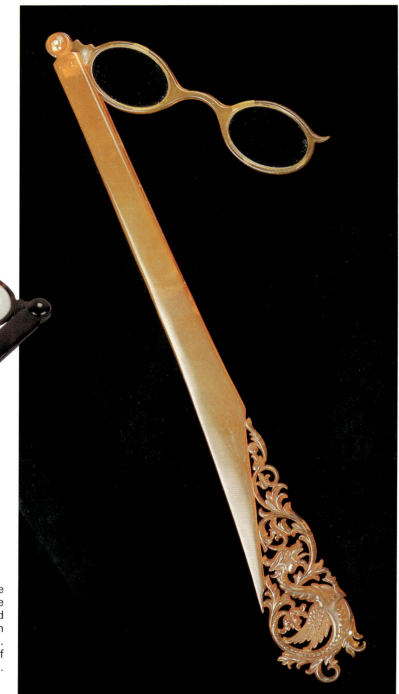

French style blonde tortoiseshell lorgnette with long handle and fantastic dragon pierced handle, c. 1890s. Courtesy of John and Valda Tull.

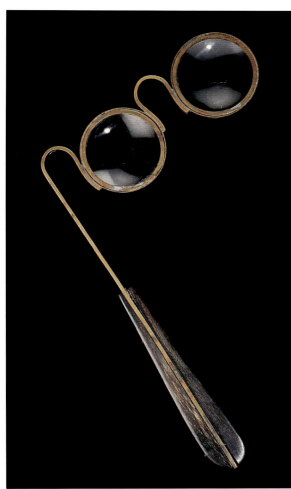
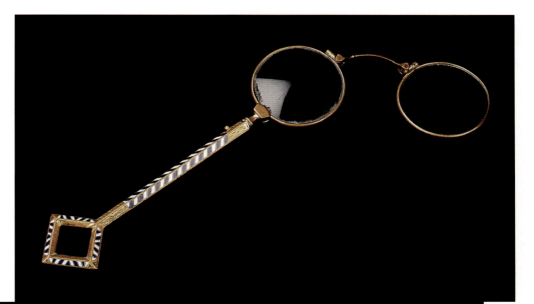

Left: Brass framed lorgnette with black bone handle marked Made in Austria Aubök (?). Courtesy of John and Valda Tull.

Right: Brass folding lorgnette with black and white enameled handle. Courtesy of John and Valda Tull.

Below: Lorgnette advertising piece with gold surface, marked Lady's Opticals. Courtesy of John and Valda Tull.

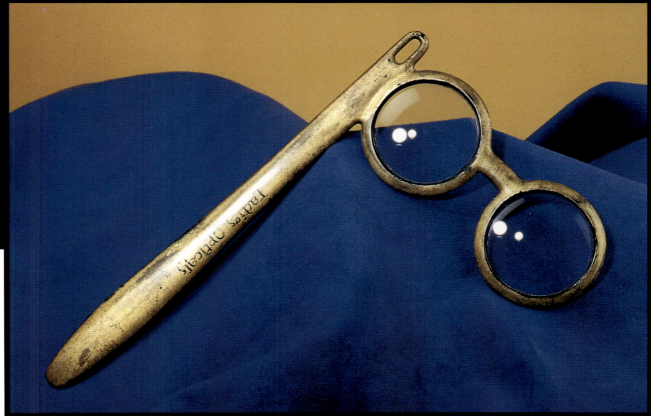

PINCE-NEZ

The term for this type of eyeglass is borrowed from French, *pince-nez* meaning literally "pinch nose." There are characteristically no temples, but a bridge or nose pads are specialized to clamp the lens frames to the bridge of the wearer's nose. Many variations on the idea were patented and made throughout the nineteenth century. An 1861 English patent (No. 389) was issued to John Braham for a bar spring of helical steel coil wire connecting the frames instead of the usual flat steel spring. An 1880 English patent (No. 5382) to Paul Goerz of Stuttgart was issued for moveable or interchangable bridges to accommodate variable facial differences of different wearers. A special bridge for pince-nez eyeglasses was patented (No. 8953) by William Curry and Joseph Fidoe Pickard of London in 1885.

The lenses of pince-nez glasses could be clear or colored, ground for single or bifocal use, or a combination of those features.

Philadelphia opticians Siegmund Lubin, John Joseph Frawley, and Albert Abraham received an English patent (No. 798) in 1887 for hinged nose rests which became very common on astigmatic pince-nez glasses. A similar design known as "Boston" were produced until the 1930s when pince-nez eyeglasses went out of fashion.

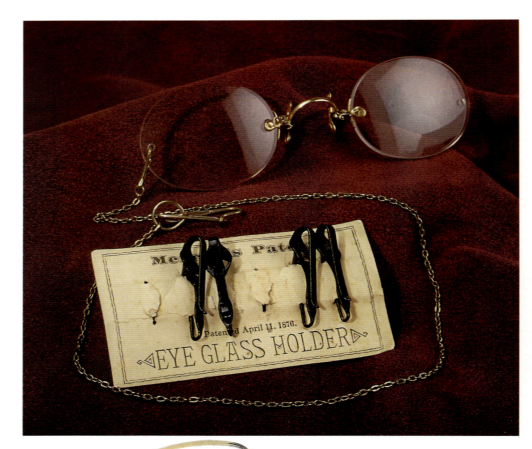

Rimless pince-nez eyeglasses with gold chain and a card of black eyeglass holder clips patented April 11, 1876. Courtesy of John and Valda Tull

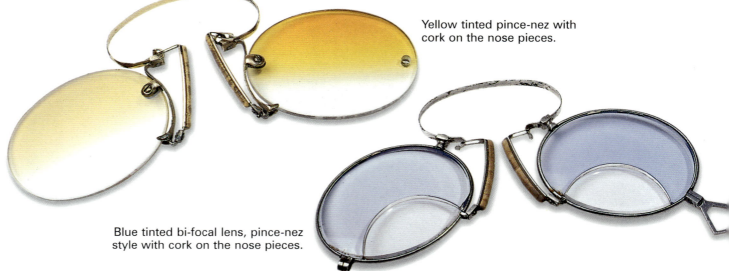

Yellow tinted pince-nez with cork on the nose pieces.

Blue tinted bi-focal lens, pince-nez style with cork on the nose pieces.

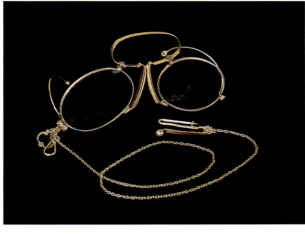

Unusual pince-nez eyeglasses with short temple pieces, large central spring, and chain with hook end. Courtesy of John and Valda Tull

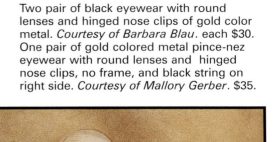

Two pair of black eyewear with round lenses and hinged nose clips of gold color metal. *Courtesy of Barbara Blau*. each $30.
One pair of gold colored metal pince-nez eyewear with round lenses and hinged nose clips, no frame, and black string on right side. *Courtesy of Mallory Gerber*. $35.

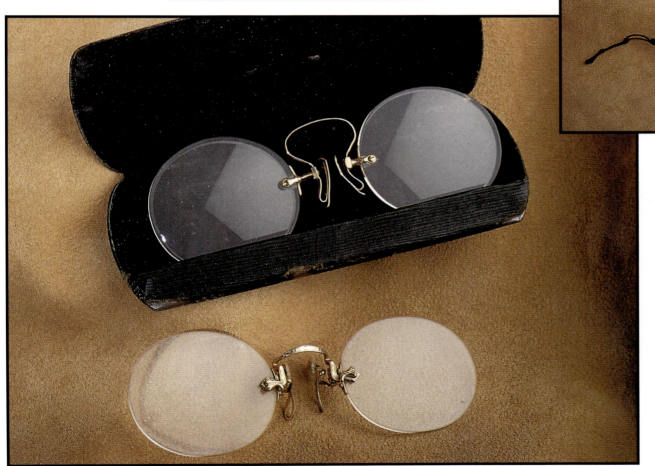

Two pair of pince-nez eyewear with round lenses, no frame, joined by gold metal nose clips, in black folding case. Courtesy of Barbara Blau.

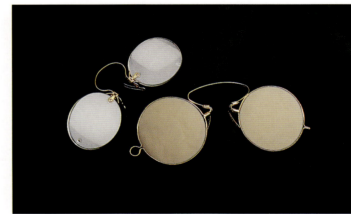

Two pair of pince-nez glasses, one with metal frames and yellow lenses. $20.
One pair without frames and hinged nose piece. *Courtesy of Barbara Blau*. $25.

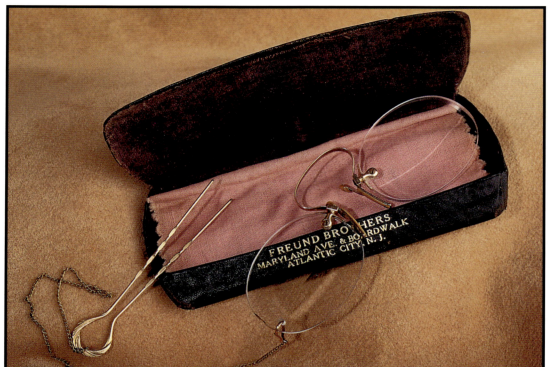

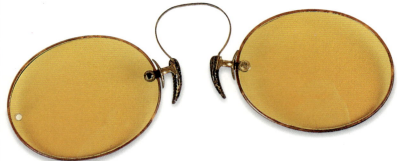

Pince-nez sunglasses with metal and celluloid frames, c. 1890. Courtesy of The Museum of Ophthalmology, Foundation of the American Academy of Ophthalmology, San Francisco

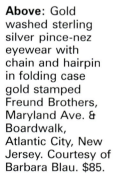

Above: Gold washed sterling silver pince-nez eyewear with chain and hairpin in folding case gold stamped Freund Brothers, Maryland Ave. & Boardwalk, Atlantic City, New Jersey. Courtesy of Barbara Blau. $85.

Right: Pince-nez tortoise framed eyeglasses with gold chain and hairpin end. Courtesy of John and Valda Tull

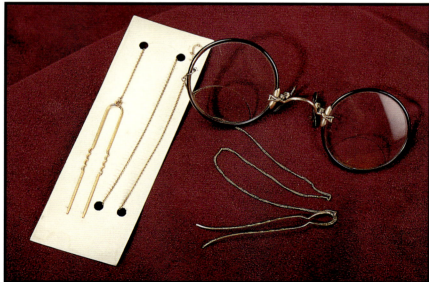

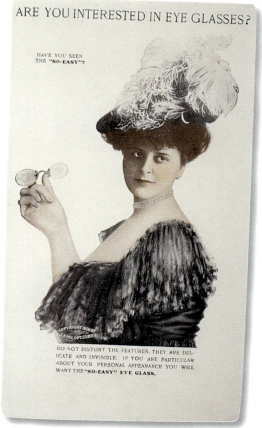

Printed paper advertisement for "So-easy" eyeglasses. Courtesy of John and Valda Tull

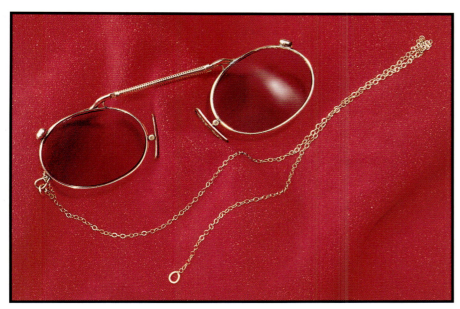

Astig clips to steady astigma correction and shaded lenses with chain.

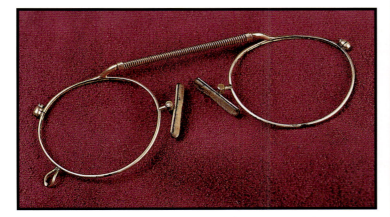

Bar-spring pince-nez glasses with wire frames, c. 1890. Courtesy of Oliver Goldsmith Eyewear Ltd.

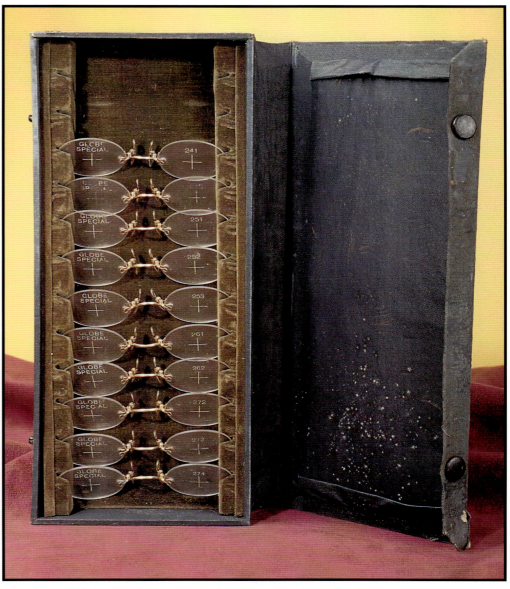

Cased set of Globe Special lenses used to determine the patient's distance between pupils. Courtesy of John and Valda Tull.

SPECIALIZED GLASSES

Eskimo shades present an essential form of eyewear specialized for protection from wind and glare in the arctic regions where they were devised. From available materials, including bone, baleen, or wood, these rigid shields were ingeniously cut by hand with a narrow slit in front of each eye to permit limited vision while protecting the face. Dating is difficult because the forms derive from styles that go back to pre-historic times. Eskimo shades were held in place with sinews or strings tied behind the head.

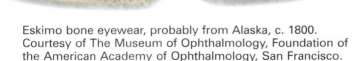

Eskimo bone eyewear, probably from Alaska, c. 1800. Courtesy of The Museum of Ophthalmology, Foundation of the American Academy of Ophthalmology, San Francisco.

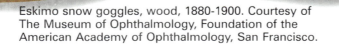

Eskimo snow goggles, wood, 1880-1900. Courtesy of The Museum of Ophthalmology, Foundation of the American Academy of Ophthalmology, San Francisco.

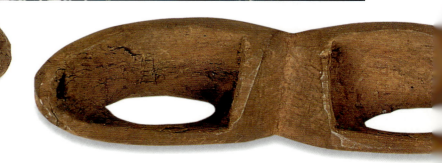

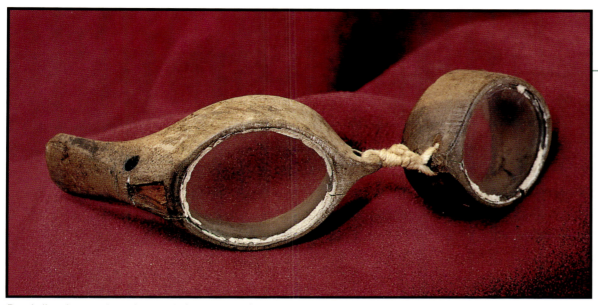

Pearl diver's wooden glasses to be strapped on. Courtesy of John and Valda Tull.

Goggles of wood with glass lenses are used by pearl divers in tropical waters today as they have been for decades, if not centuries.

Coal cinders, smoke, and wind provided hazards to railroad personnel as well as passengers in open cars and an opportunity to protect their eyes was met with the development of specialized eyewear. In the second half of the nineteenth century, railroad eyeglasses with D-shaped lenses of colored glass and folding side lenses were made in large numbers. Some varieties had removable temples (as shown) and they typically came with a carrying box of wood or cardboard.

Left & below: Sunglasses and case. Glass, metal, plastic; case, wood, leather, silk, and velvet. France, c. 1850-75. Courtesy of The Museum of Ophthalmology, Foundation of the American Academy of Ophthalmology, San Francisco.

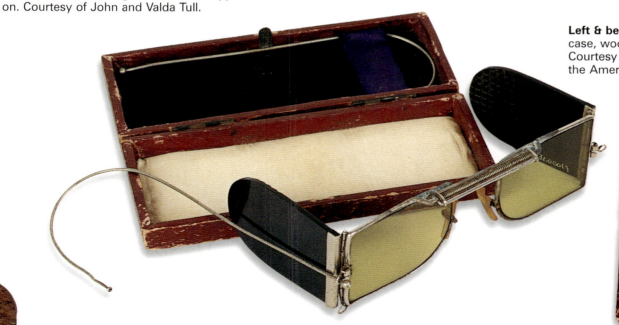

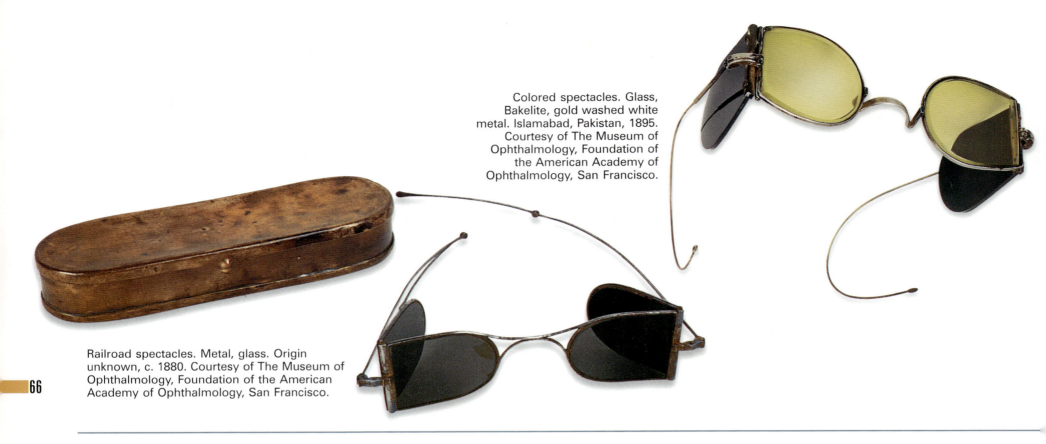

Colored spectacles. Glass, Bakelite, gold washed white metal. Islamabad, Pakistan, 1895. Courtesy of The Museum of Ophthalmology, Foundation of the American Academy of Ophthalmology, San Francisco.

Railroad spectacles. Metal, glass. Origin unknown, c. 1880. Courtesy of The Museum of Ophthalmology, Foundation of the American Academy of Ophthalmology, San Francisco.

An 1888 English patent (No. 6059) was issued to George Paxton and Willaim Curry for goggles with wire gauze cups to be worn as pince-nez glasses "for the protection of the eyes against the sun and wind, and adapted to the bridge of our pince-nez." And in 1893, Robert Purdom and Henry Stokes of Birmingham patented (No. 14648) improved eye protectors "by the addition of metal supports connecting the upper and lower rims forming the binding of the gauze cups and D-shaped gauze's. The metal supports may be cupped or raised to give them additional strength." This improvement was widely used.

Another design for railroad personnel comprises metal mesh goggles around oval, clear or blue glass lenses and a fastening cord to go around the head. These remain in quite large numbers today.

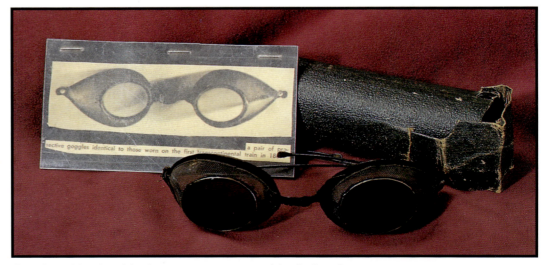

Goggles with wire sides in green canvas case, identical to those worn on the first transcontinental train in 1869. Courtesy of John and Valda Tull

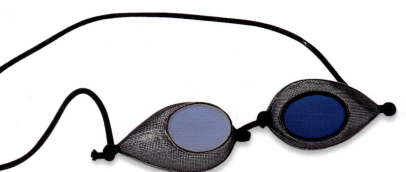

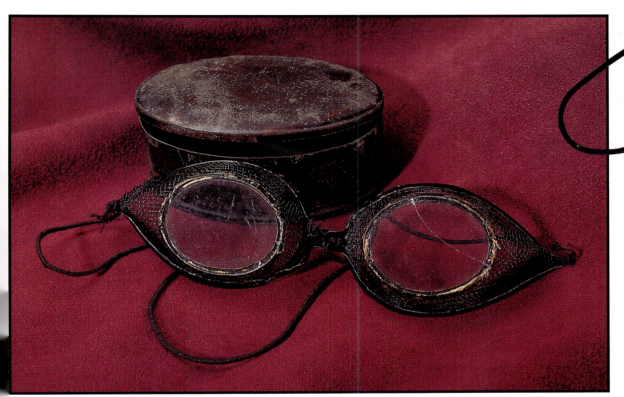

Above: Railroad goggles. Glass, metal, rope (not original). Blue lenses with wire mesh side screens. USA, 1880-1900. Courtesy of The Museum of Ophthalmology, Foundation of the American Academy of Ophthalmology, San Francisco.

Left: Railroad goggles with string attachment and wire screen sides, in small oval tin case. Courtesy of John and Valda Tull

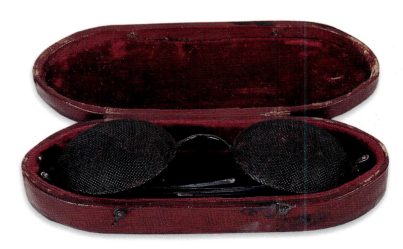

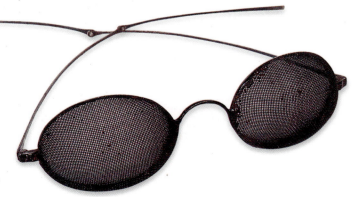

Protective eyewear and case. Wire mesh convex screens. Metal, leather; metal, velvet. L.P. Cutts, England. c. 1870. Courtesy of The Museum of Ophthalmology, Foundation of the American Academy of Ophthalmology, San Francisco.

Eyeglasses from the late nineteenth century specialized for use while gunning have frosted and tinted glass lenses, usually in gray or amber shades, with a defined clear circle in front of the eyes' pupils. The supposition seems to have been that this design caused the hunter to focus carefully on the target without peripheral distraction. John Braham was granted an English patent (No. 389) in 1861 for his design which featured a small eye hole in the center of an opaque lens "immediately in front of the pupil of the eye" for rifle shooting and other puroposes where great steadiness of sight is required. In 1892, an English patent (No. 15745) was granted to Matthew Mullineux, a cartridge maker from Manchester, England, for "frames of orthoptics used in shooting." In his design, a leather-lined nose cap of thin sheet metal "is fixed on the wire frame in such a position that it fits the nose exactly keeping the orthoptic [lenses] vertical when the marksman is in position."

A unique design for pivoting eyeglasses specialized for playing billiards was patented (No. 16123) in 1895 by William Berthold Ihne of Liverpool.

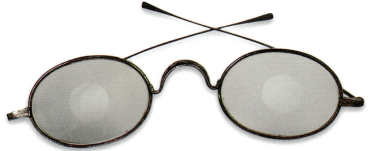

Above: Gunning glasses. Metal, glass. Used to increase accuracy in marksmanship. c. 1879-80. Courtesy of The Museum of Ophthalmology, Foundation of the American Academy of Ophthalmology, San Francisco.

Right: Gunning glasses. Steel. Amber lenses. United States, c. 1885. Courtesy of The Museum of Ophthalmology, Foundation of the American Academy of Ophthalmology, San Francisco.

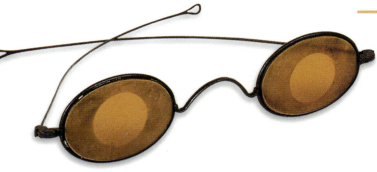

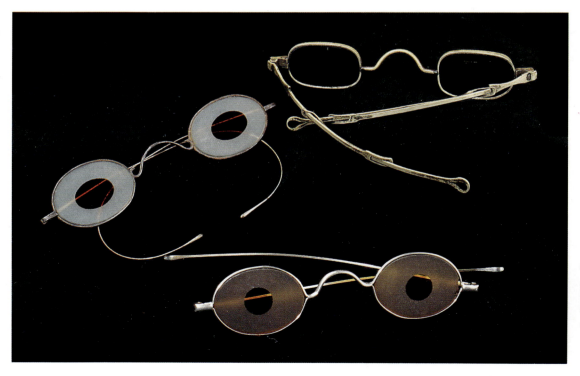

Three gunning glasses with yellow, blue, and pink coloring. Courtesy of John and Valda Tull.

20 TH CENTURY

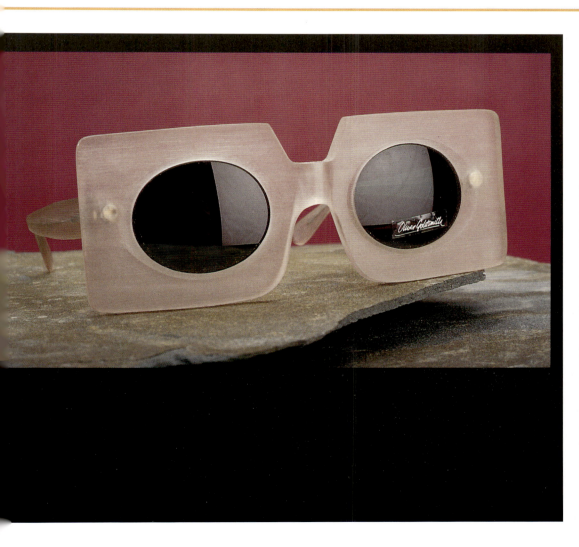

The twentieth century as a whole has been a time of gradual and dramatic change in the eyewear business, in fact the business has become an industry. Along with progress in lens acuity and frame shapes, sunglasses became popular accessories for both men and women in both plain and prescription strength. Beginning in the 1950s, eyeglasses began to be coordinated with clothing in their colors and ornamentation. In the 1960s, the fashion of wearing eyeglasses began to be desirable for people with perfect vision as well as people who needed corrective lenses. Men and women alike were shown in advertisements for many consumer goods to be wearing different regular glasses and sunglasses for each activity. This fashion trend, coupled with the popularity of sunglasses to hide the faces of celebrity entertainers, caused exotic and trendy styles of frames to be made and avidly worn in the 1970s and 1980s. Mature socialites and ingenues alike preferred to be seen wearing exotic sunglasses day and night for casual and formal events. As lighter weight lenses and frame materials were developed, they were quickly utilized in the eyewear field. The most conservative as well as the most original clothing designers worldwide showed eyeglasses and sunglasses with their new lines of clothing in the 1990s, and many of them licensed eyewear to sell along with their clothes. Their coordinated ensembles, including their own styles of eyewear, received mass-media promotion.

EARLY 20TH CENTURY

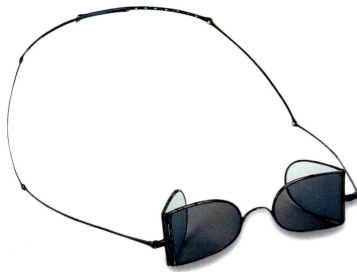

Colored spectacles. Glass, brass. Amber lenses. 1900-1909. Courtesy of The Museum of Ophthalmology, Foundation of the American Academy of Ophthalmology, San Francisco.

Spectacles, glass and blued steel. Temple pieces make up a headband with adjustable links. c. 1900. Courtesy of The Museum of Ophthalmology, Foundation of the American Academy of Ophthalmology, San Francisco.

Spectacles. Rimless. Glass, gold. c. 1905. Courtesy of The Museum of Ophthalmology, Foundation of the American Academy of Ophthalmology, San Francisco.

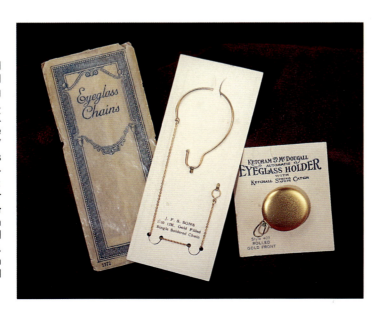

Left: printed paper card advertising eyeglass chains. Center: "1/10 12K gold filled single soldered chain" by J. F. S. Sons with ear attachment. Right: Eyeglass holder by Ketcham & McDougall with "rolled gold front," c.1900. Courtesy of John and Valda Tull

In the early decades of the twentieth century, small and independent opticians continued to make eyeglasses by hand and with limited mechanical means. Salesmen for the manufacturers went door to door to jewelry stores selling lenses and frames separately. The popular use of ear hooks to secure a chain attached to glasses was based on an English patent (No. 20652) issued in 1894 to David Roberts of Carnarvonshire.

Folding eyeglass styles became popular and common after the turn of the century. Not new in design, folding eyeglasses had been improved throughout the nineteenth century with patents for specialized catches (1887, No. 2020, to Charles Heath) and bridges (1887, No. 9202, to C. W. Taylor). Walter W. Whitehouse received an English patent (No. 18712) in 1892 for an "improved folding eyeglass" with a pivoting bridge that "allows the eyeglass to be folded, which is an advantage especially when they are fitted with astigmatic lenses."

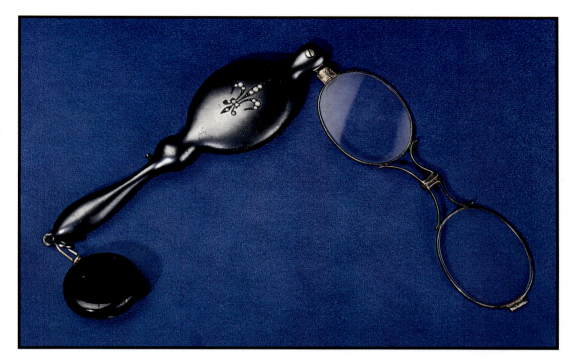

Steel folding lorgnette with attached pin marked Ketcham & McDougall, Pat. Feb. 24, 1903, New York, with fleur-de-lis pearl inlay. Courtesy of John and Valda Tull.

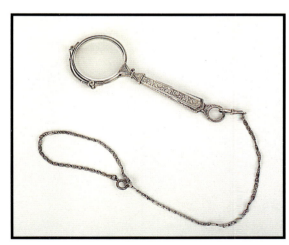

Lorgnette. Glass, sterling silver. Russia, c. 1910. Wrist chain. Courtesy of The Museum of Ophthalmology, Foundation of the American Academy of Ophthalmology, San Francisco.

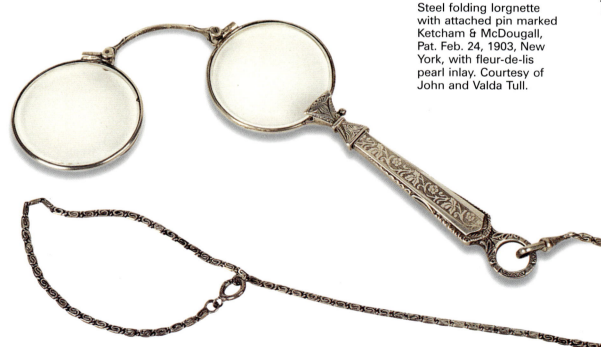

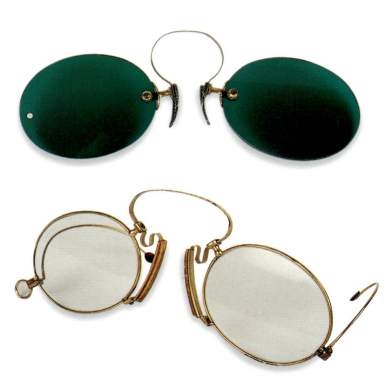

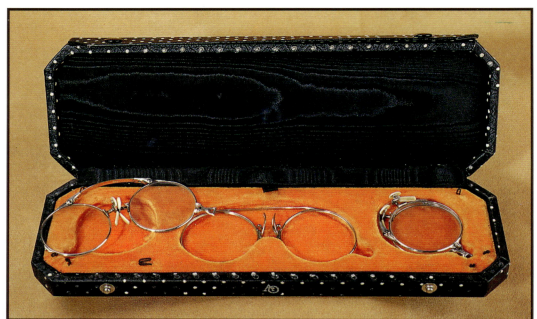

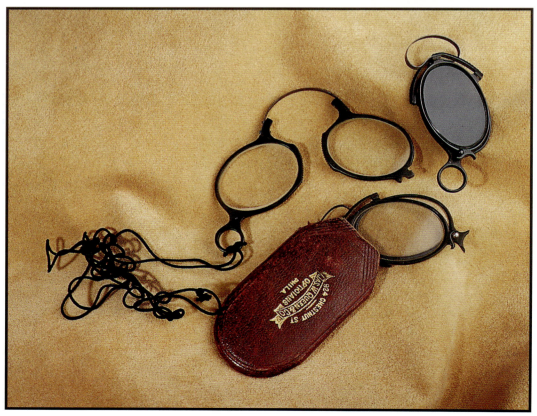

Top left: Pince-nez glasses. Glass, steel or brass fittings. Green lenses. c. 1910. Courtesy of The Museum of Ophthalmology, Foundation of the American Academy of Ophthalmology, San Francisco.

Above: Pince-nez glasses. Gold, glass. c. 1910. Courtesy of The Museum of Ophthalmology, Foundation of the American Academy of Ophthalmology, San Francisco.

Top right: Black cased sales kit for Oxford style pince-nez glasses with two folding styles and one not folding. Courtesy of John and Valda Tull.

Right: Folding black gutta percha eyewear with original brown leather case stamped in gold Jas. W. Owen & Co. Opticians, 9224 Chestnut St., Philadelphia. Courtesy of Mallory Gerber. $45.

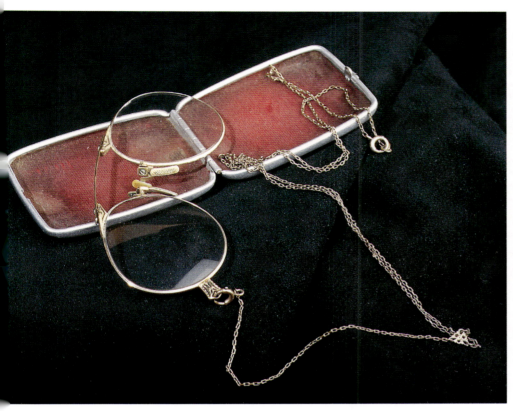

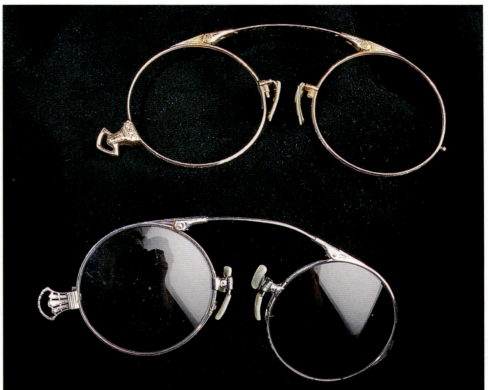

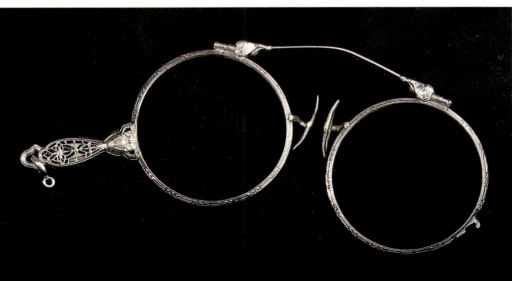

Above left: Folding eyewear of gold colored metal frames with black enamel stripes and gold chain, in metal case. Courtesy of Barbara Blau. $95.

Above right: Folding pince-nez eyewear with patterned silver frame and filigree handle, marked USA. Courtesy of Barbara Blau. $75.

Left: Two pair of folding pince-nez glasses, one with gold filled frame. $35.
Other with patterned silver frame. Courtesy of Barbara Blau. $65.

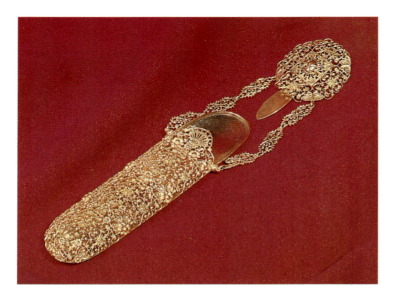

Left: Gilt chatelaine eyeglass case of filigree work.

Below: English sterling chatelaine of openwork with eyeglass case suspended on chains. Courtesy of John and Valda Tull.

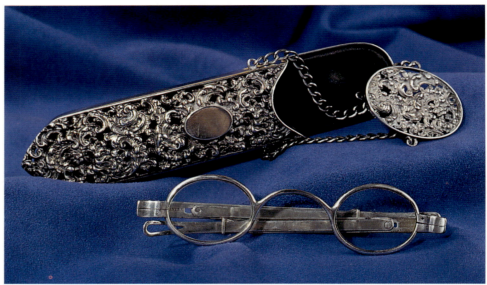

Improvements in eyeglass cases also were forthcoming. In 1895, George Hall, a jeweler from Birmingham, received a patent (No. 11236) for a chateleine case with additional compartments for a penholder and pencil. These styles continued to be fashionable until the 1920s.

Steel rim frame eye glasses and a shagreen case with open end and silver edge with English hallmarks, c. 1913. Oliver Goldsmith Eyewear Ltd.

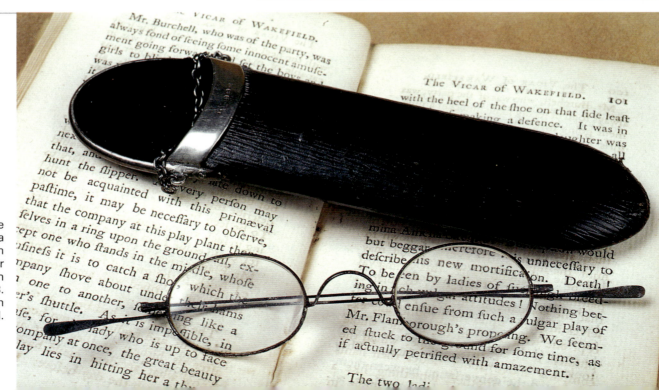

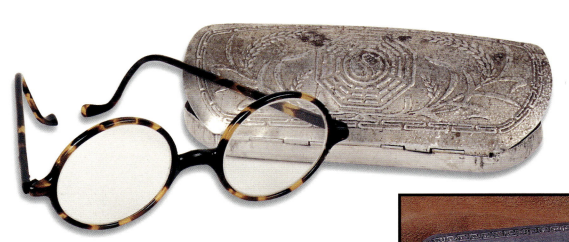

Above: Spectacles and case. Glass, plastic. Aluminum case. China?, c. 1915. Courtesy of The Museum of Ophthalmology, Foundation of the American Academy of Ophthalmology, San Francisco.

Right: Aluminum case from a Dublin maker and silver hallmarked glasses.

During the first World War, the frightening use of poison gas and the use of open cockpit airplanes caused specialized eyewear to be developed to protect people from the effects of their respective exposure.

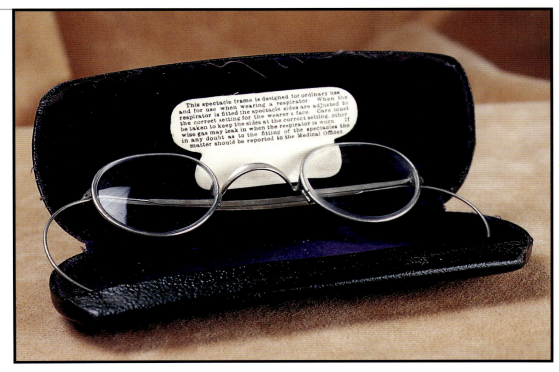

Wire rim eye glasses designed to be worn when wearing a respirator, c. 1915. Oliver Goldsmith Eyewear Ltd.

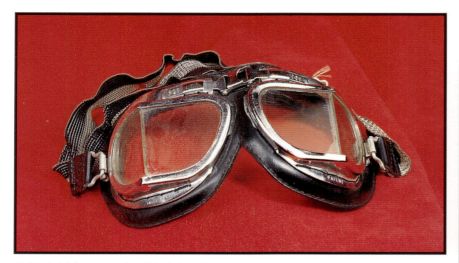

Pair of driving goggles, black leather and chrome around two-piece glass lenses, marked Made in England. Courtesy of Helaine Fendelman.

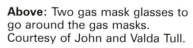

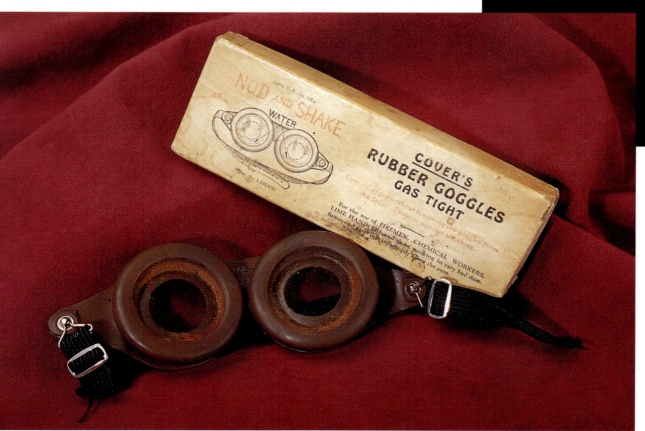

Above: Two gas mask glasses to go around the gas masks. Courtesy of John and Valda Tull.

Left: Cover's Rubber Goggles with gas tight seal for use by firemen, chemical workers, and lime handlers to avoid dust. Courtesy of John and Valda Tull.

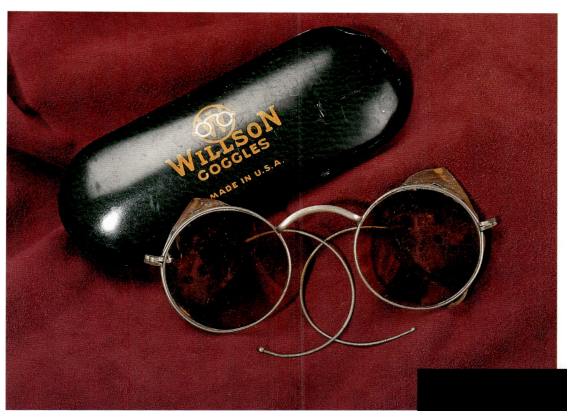

Left: Willson Goggles of Reading, Pa. with metal frames and leather sides, in green painted tin case. Courtesy of John and Valda Tull.

Below: A master's small pair of glasses with exquisite work to demonstrate proficient skill. Courtesy of John and Valda Tull.

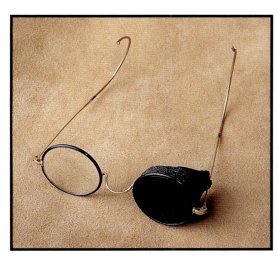

Amblyopia (lazy eye) child's glasses with one lens blocked, gold bridge and ear pieces.

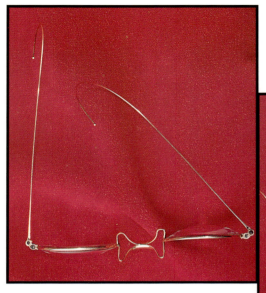
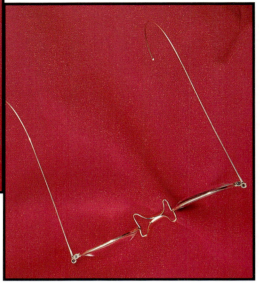

Unusual gold glasses for someone who has had cataract surgery in one eye. The arms swing both ways to adjust for near- and farsighted correction. The nose piece is constructed to work from both sides.

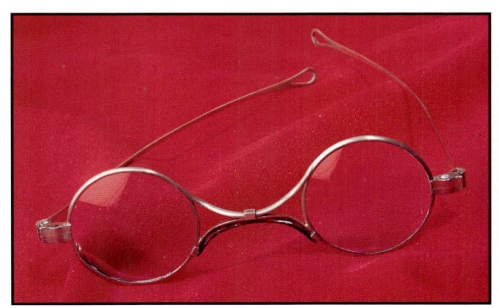

Another unusual pair for a person who has had cataract surgery. The lenses are tinted blue and the steel frames can be worn upside down.

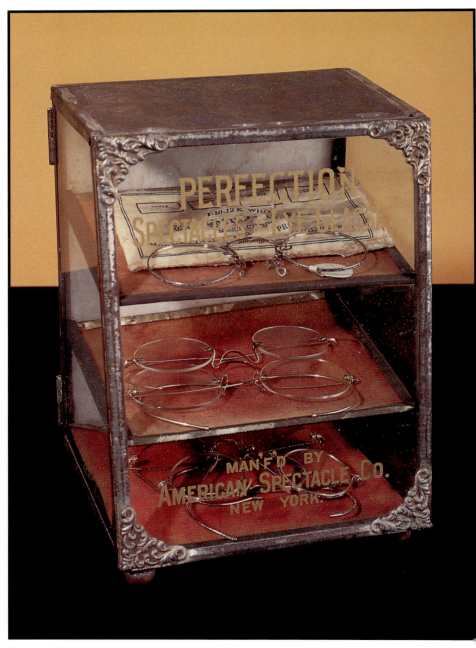

Tin and glass counter display, c. early 20th century, front marked Perfection Spectacles & Eye Glasses Man'f'd by American Spectacle Co., New York. Courtesy of John and Valda Tull.

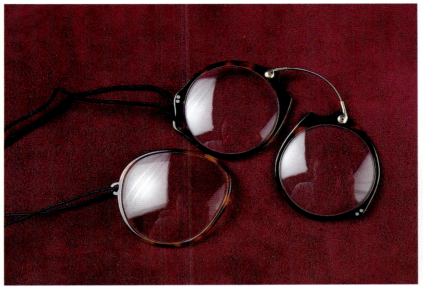

Eyewear was pretty much a mundane affair in the roaring 1920s, for visually impaired people, many of whom would rather not wear their glasses in public. Tortoiseshell frames, both hand- and machine-made, were preferred as opposed to metal frames which were considered "old fashioned."

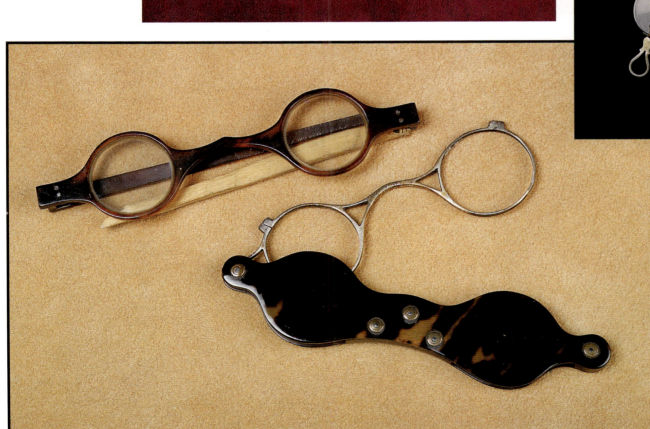

Above left: Tortoiseshell pince-nez eyeglasses with cord and a tortoiseshell monocle with cord, c. 1920s. Oliver Goldsmith Eyewear Ltd.

Above: Pince-nez glasses and case marked E. A. Barnitz & Son Jewelers, York, Penna., c. 1920s. Courtesy of John and Valda Tull.

Left: Folding tortoiseshell lorgnette with steel rims. And small pair of tortoiseshell frames with ground lenses, c. 1920. Oliver Goldsmith Eyewear Ltd.

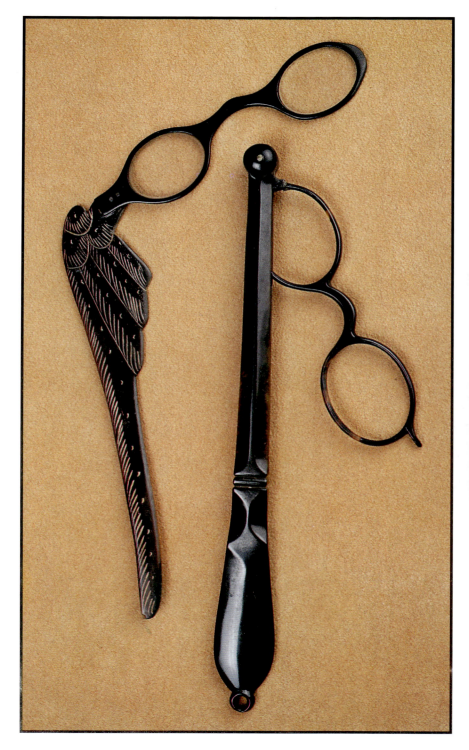

Left: Pair of tortoiseshell lorgnette with hinged handle, and a pair of horn lorgnette with immovable handle, c. 1920s. Oliver Goldsmith Eyewear Ltd.

Below: Frame of 14k gold with round lenses in a folding case marked Orthogon Lenses. Courtesy of Aida's Antiques. $150.

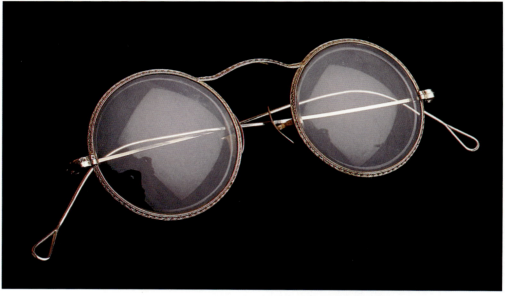

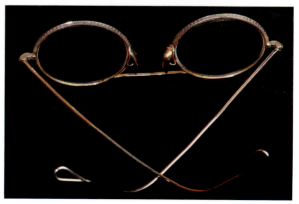

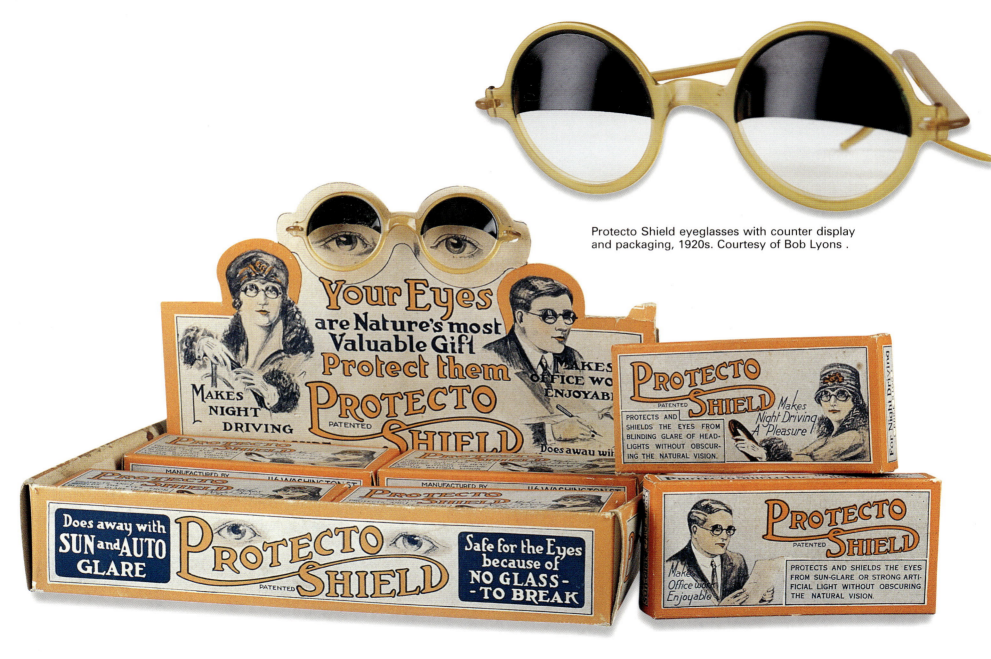

Protecto Shield eyeglasses with counter display and packaging, 1920s. Courtesy of Bob Lyons.

81

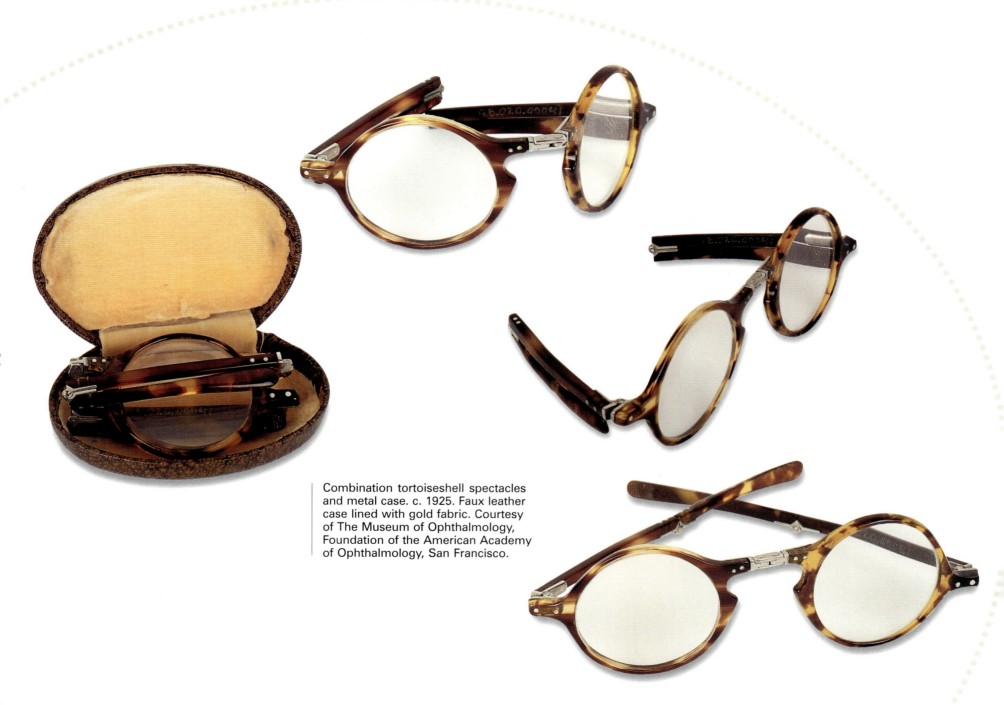

Combination tortoiseshell spectacles and metal case. c. 1925. Faux leather case lined with gold fabric. Courtesy of The Museum of Ophthalmology, Foundation of the American Academy of Ophthalmology, San Francisco.

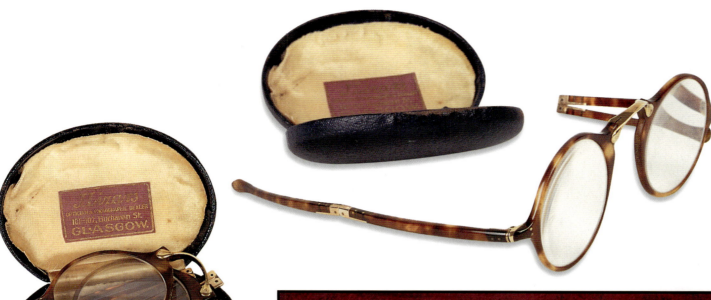

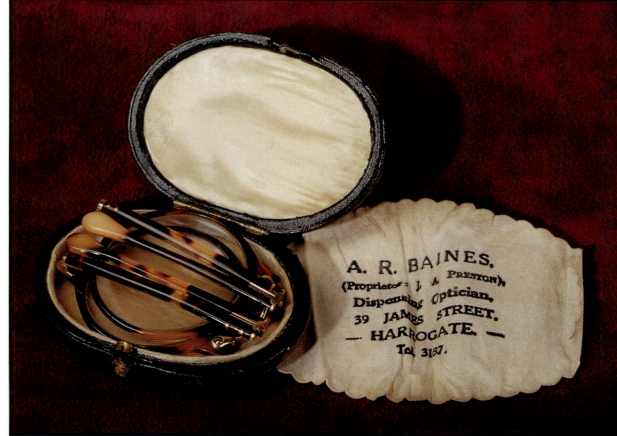

Above: Spectacles. Tortoiseshell, gold. J. Lizars, Optician. Glasgow, Scotland, c. 1925. Leather-covered steel case. Courtesy of The Museum of Ophthalmology, Foundation of the American Academy of Ophthalmology, San Francisco.

Right: Tortoiseshell folding glasses in case with cleaning cloth printed A. R. Binnes, Harrogate. Courtesy of John and Valda Tull.

The London-based maker of hand-cut tortoiseshell eyeglass frames Oliver Goldsmith began in 1926 to serve the growing market for eyeglasses. Innovative in materials as well as designs, this firm introduced by 1928 frames of colored Erinoid plastics (the Chelsea Art spectacle) and a new hinge to fit inside the frame to give a more sleek appearance (the Prince spectacle). Soon thereafter Oliver Goldsmith introduced the first flesh-colored frames (Dawn) which remained in production for many years.

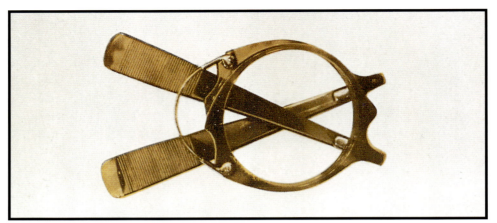

Tortoiseshell eyeglasses, 1928, "Pocket." Oliver Goldsmith Eyewear Ltd.

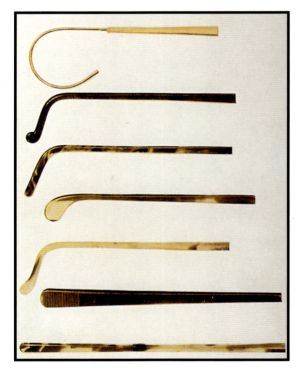

Tortoiseshell eyeglasses, 1928, showing seven ear pieces. Oliver Goldsmith Eyewear Ltd.

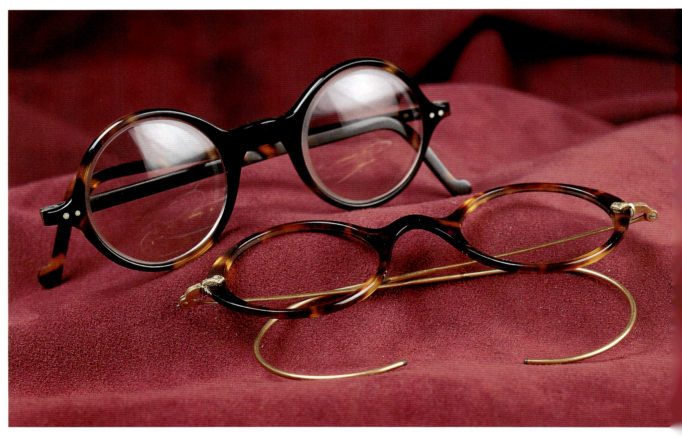

Two pair of tortoiseshell eyeglasses, c. 1920s. Oliver Goldsmith Eyewear Ltd.

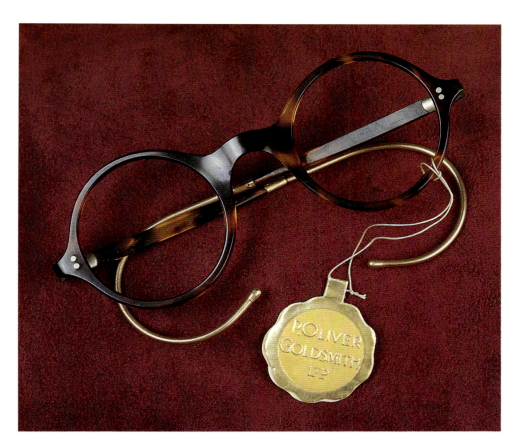

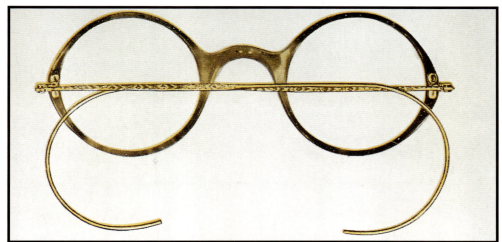

Above left: Tortoiseshell eyeglasses, c. 1920s. P. Oliver Goldsmith, Ltd.

Above Right: Tortoiseshell eyeglasses, 1928, "Portsmouth." Oliver Goldsmith Eyewear Ltd.

Below left: Tortoiseshell eyeglasses, 1928, "Bull Dog." Oliver Goldsmith Eyewear Ltd.

Below right: Tortoiseshell eyeglasses, 1928, "Adelaide." Oliver Goldsmith Eyewear Ltd.

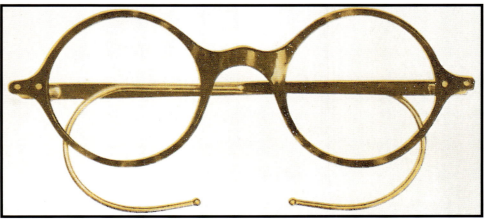

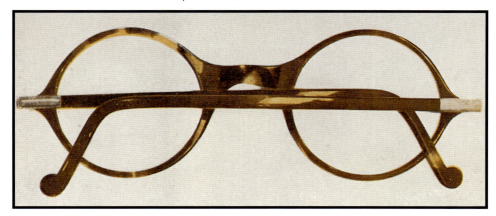

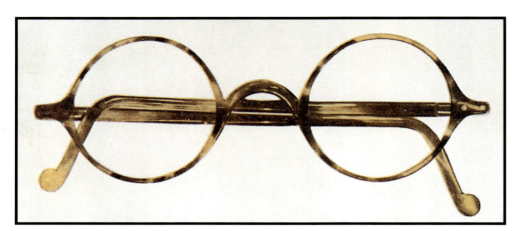

Tortoiseshell eyeglasses, 1928, "Elfin."
Oliver Goldsmith Eyewear Ltd.

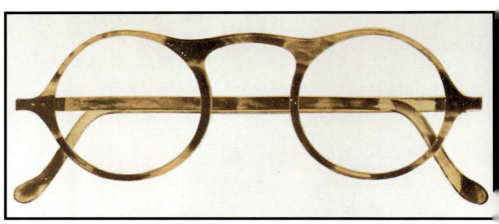

Tortoiseshell eyeglasses, 1928, "Padishell."
Oliver Goldsmith Eyewear Ltd.

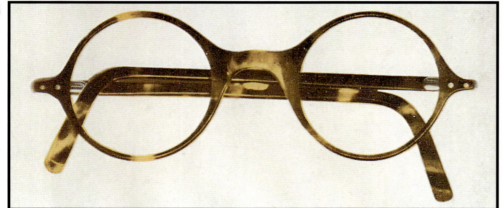

Tortoiseshell eyeglasses, 1928, "Poland."
Oliver Goldsmith Eyewear Ltd.

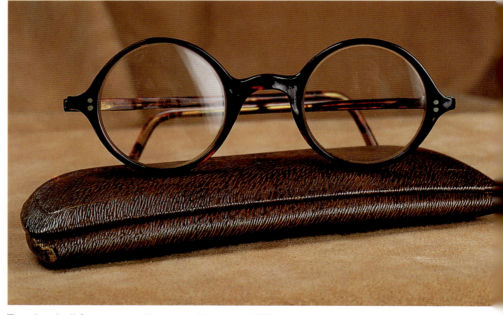

Tortoiseshell frame eye glasses and case, c. 1920s.
Oliver Goldsmith Eyewear Ltd.

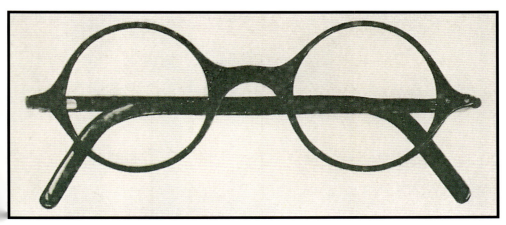

Tortoiseshell eyeglasses, 1928, "Chelsea Art," made from colorful Erinoid plastic. Oliver Goldsmith Eyewear Ltd.

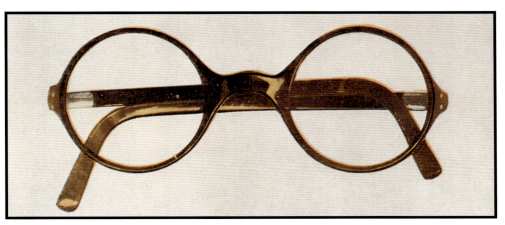

Tortoiseshell eyeglasses, 1928, "Prince," with inside hinge. Oliver Goldsmith Eyewear Ltd

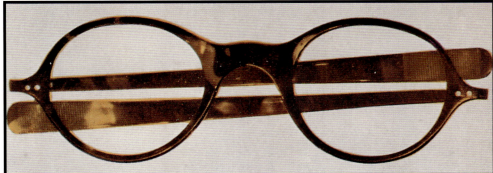

Tortoiseshell eyeglasses, 1928, "Library." Oliver Goldsmith Eyewear Ltd.

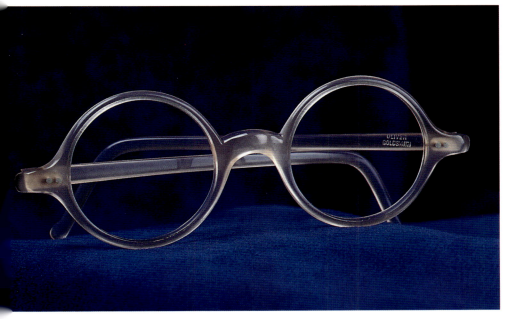

The first flesh-colored plastic frame called Dawn, as it was the dawn of a new era in eyewear, c. 1940. Oliver Goldsmith Eyewear Ltd.

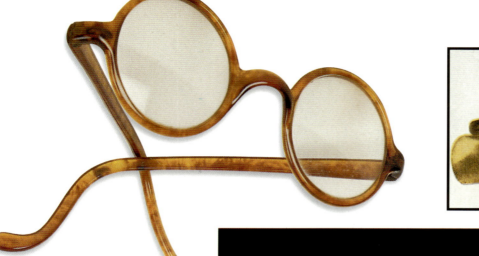
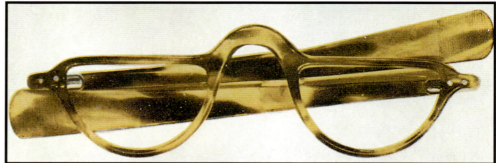
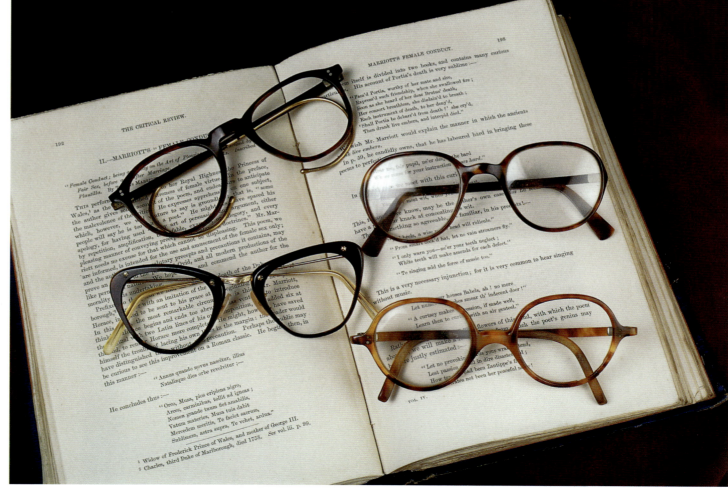

Above: Eyeglasses with light brown tortoiseshell frames, c. 1930-1940. Courtesy of The Museum of Ophthalmology, Foundation of the American Academy of Ophthalmology, San Francisco.

Above right: Tortoiseshell eyeglasses, 1928, "Artist." Oliver Goldsmith Eyewear Ltd.

Right: Four pair of tortoiseshell glasses, c. 1920s. Oliver Goldsmith Eyewear Ltd.

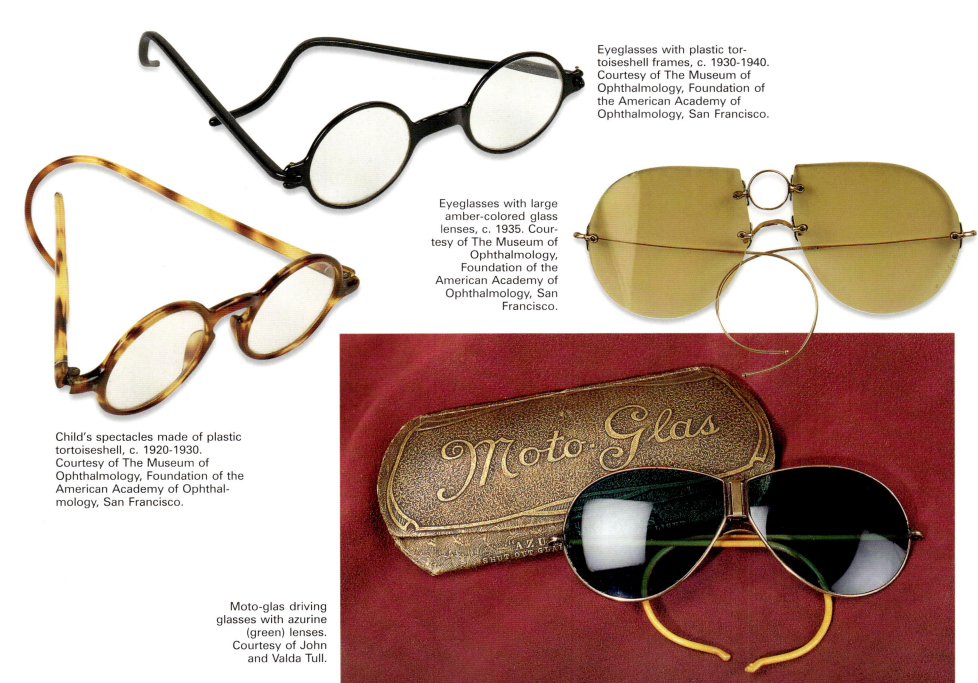

Eyeglasses with plastic tortoiseshell frames, c. 1930-1940. Courtesy of The Museum of Ophthalmology, Foundation of the American Academy of Ophthalmology, San Francisco.

Eyeglasses with large amber-colored glass lenses, c. 1935. Courtesy of The Museum of Ophthalmology, Foundation of the American Academy of Ophthalmology, San Francisco.

Child's spectacles made of plastic tortoiseshell, c. 1920-1930. Courtesy of The Museum of Ophthalmology, Foundation of the American Academy of Ophthalmology, San Francisco.

Moto-glas driving glasses with azurine (green) lenses. Courtesy of John and Valda Tull.

The widespread use of rhinestones came to women's popular jewelry in the 1930s and they were incorporated into designs for eyewear as well. The folding lorgnette/dress clip style shown is an example of beautiful quality, hand-set eyewear that is truly also an item of jewelry.

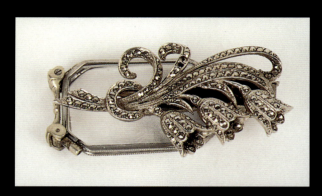

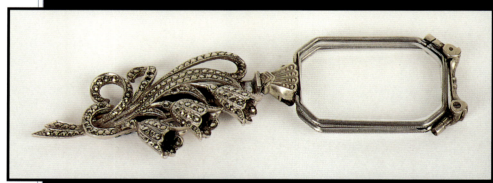

Lorgnette with marcasite ornament. United States, c. 1930. Courtesy of The Museum of Ophthalmology, Foundation of the American Academy of Ophthalmology, San Francisco.

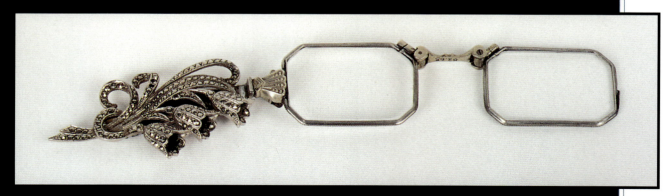

MID-TWENTIETH CENTURY

Optical shops were established in every small town by the 1940s as the population grew and eyeglasses became a standard vision aid for a larger segment of the population. People who wore eyeglasses in rural areas often boxed the glasses up in sturdy wooden cartons and sent them for repair through the postal system to their optometrist, optician, or manufacturer.

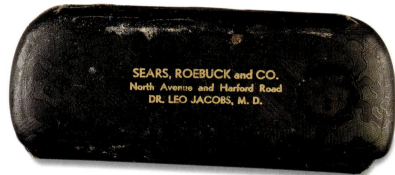

Hard case with hinged lid inscribed "Sears Roebuck and Co., Dr. Leo Jacobs, M.D."

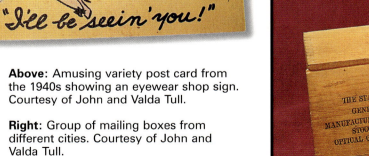

Above: Amusing variety post card from the 1940s showing an eyewear shop sign. Courtesy of John and Valda Tull.

Right: Group of mailing boxes from different cities. Courtesy of John and Valda Tull.

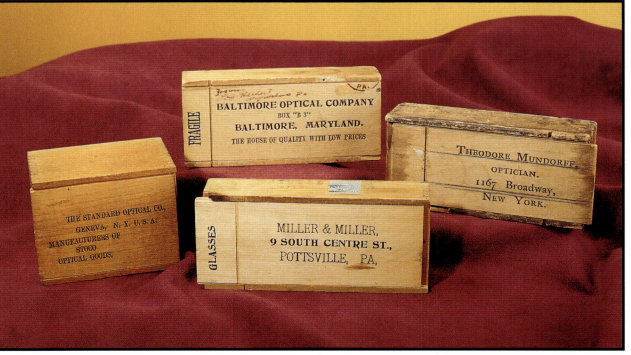

Steel frames around small rectangular lenses and sliding earpieces marked "18" (focal point). The hard and hinged case is stamped in gold D. W. Peel Optometrist Haverhill, Massachusetts. Courtesy of Bill Drucker.

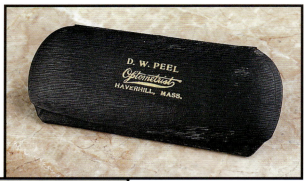

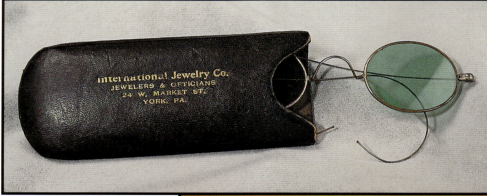

International Jewelry Co. Jewelers & Opticians 24 West Market St. York, Pa. Courtesy of John and Valda Tull.

Group of mailing boxes from different cities. Courtesy of John and Valda Tull

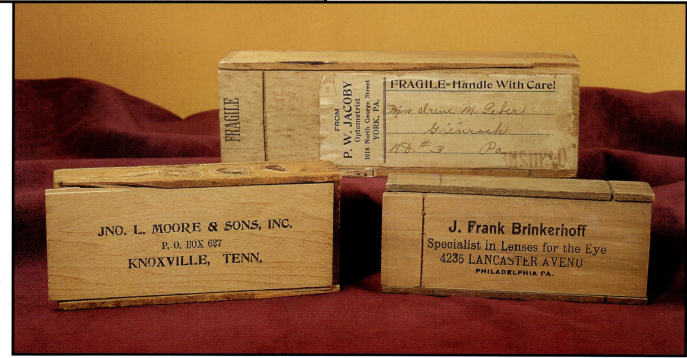

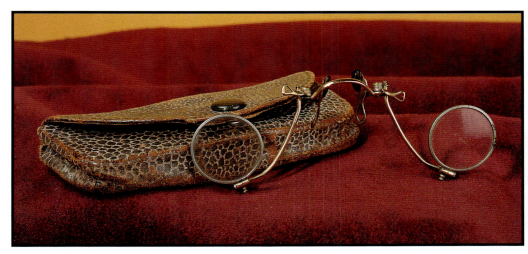

Supplementary magnifying lenses to attach to eyeglasses, with shagreen case. *Courtesy of John and Valda Tull*

Specialty glasses were constantly improved and modified for individual applications from additional clip-on lenses for jewelers and clock makers to goggles for aviators and welders. Tinted glass eyeglasses were more widely available as inexpensive sunglasses by the late 1940s.

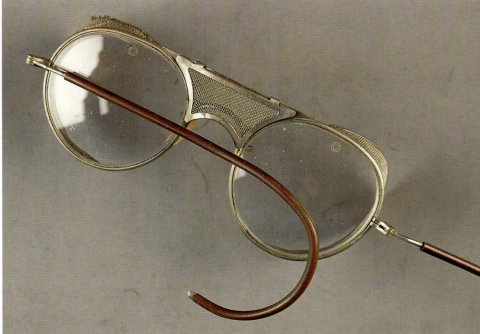

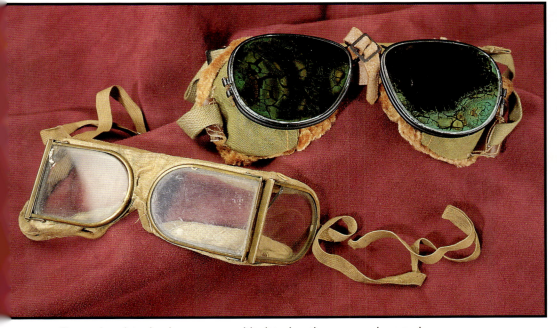

Two pair aviator's glasses, one with deteriorating green glass and canvas frames and one with front and side lenses and canvas frames with elastic bands. Courtesy of John and Valda Tull.

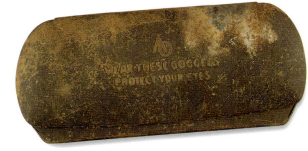

Above: American Optical safety glasses.

Left: Metal case marked A O (American Optical) Wear these Goggles Protect your eyes. Private collection.

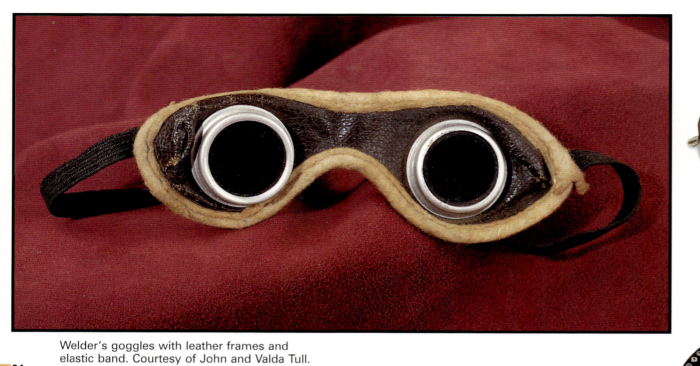

Welder's goggles with leather frames and elastic band. Courtesy of John and Valda Tull.

One of the earliest examples of "cheap" sunglasses. Metal and plastic. c. 1940. Courtesy of The Museum of Ophthalmology, Foundation of the American Academy of Ophthalmology, San Francisco.

Folding lorgnette. Plastic, rhinestones. Hong Kong, c. 1940. Courtesy of The Museum of Ophthalmology, Foundation of the American Academy of Ophthalmology, San Francisco.

Lorgnette. Plastic, rhinestones, glass. c. 1930s-50s. Courtesy of The Museum of Ophthalmology, Foundation of the American Academy of Ophthalmology, San Francisco.

Brown layered eyewear marked American Optical "Sea Mist," True Color CN86T. Courtesy of Barbara Blau.

Eyeglass maker Oliver Goldsmith of London designed and handmade new styles of sunglasses to coordinate with clothing in the fashion world. He advertised them in the 1950s in popular magazines such as *Vogue*, *Tatler*, and *Harper & Queen*. Department stores bought the sunglasses readily and sold them to an enthusiastic public. Many eyeglass makers worldwide made new designs for both clear and tinted glass spectacles available in a wide variety of plastics and metals at very competitive prices. Many styles became ornamented with jewel-like embellishments and inserts, and the public loved them.

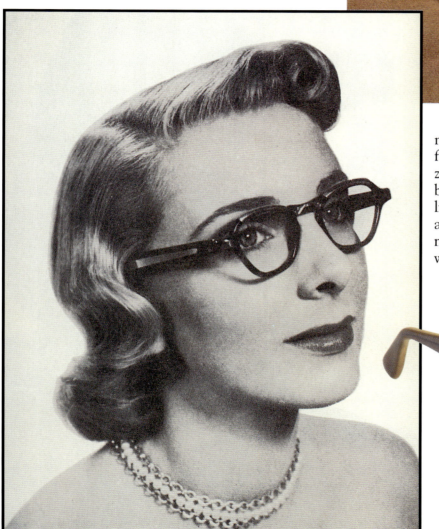

Sunglasses. Plastic, glass, rhinestones. c. 1950. Courtesy of The Museum of Ophthalmology, Foundation of the American Academy of Ophthalmology, San Francisco.

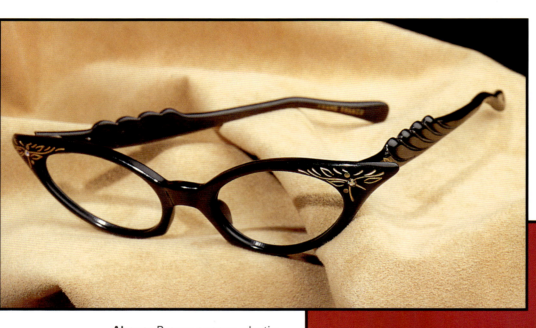

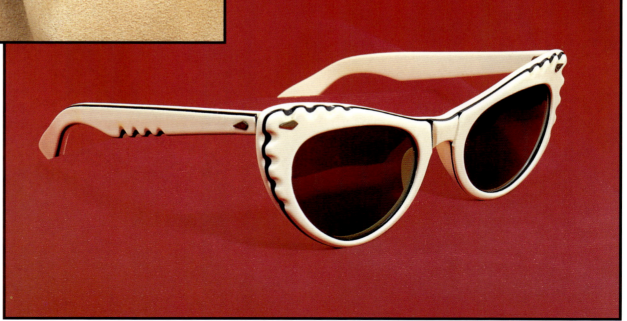

Sunglasses. Plastic, prescription lenses, accented with rhinestones. Frfund Brothers, France, c. 1950. Courtesy of The Museum of Ophthalmology, Foundation of the American Academy of Ophthalmology, San Francisco.

Above: Brown opaque plastic frames with gold incised and rhinestone decorated corners, marked Frame France. Courtesy of Aida's Antiques.

Right: Sunglasses. White plastic frames with black detailing and ruffled corners, marked Calobar CC31-50. Courtesy of Helaine Fendelman.

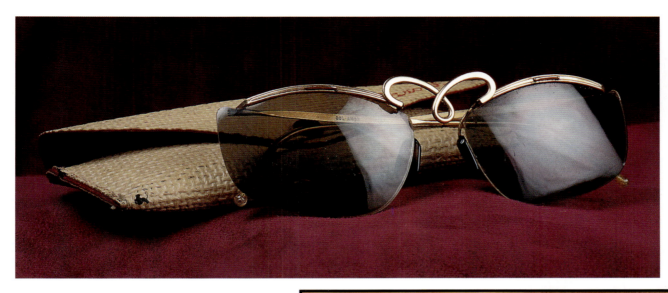

Polaroid plastic tinted lenses, c. 1950s. Courtesy of Oliver Goldsmith Eyewear Ltd.

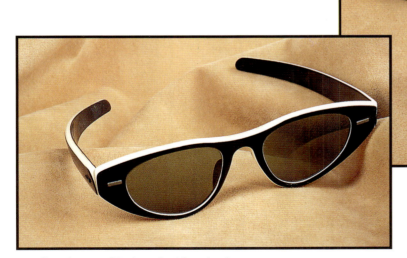

Sunglasses. Black and white plastic frames marked Cool Ray Emeraldlite. Courtesy of Helaine Fendelman.

Above: Folding metal-rim frames with hinged and rhinestone decorated tinted visor and lenses, with hard plastic case marked D. Pat. No. 132011, K.K. Spectacle Co. Made in Japan. Courtesy of Helaine Fendelman.

Right: Black plastic frames with silver and gold corner pieces, marked USA Sherman. Courtesy of Aida's Antiques.

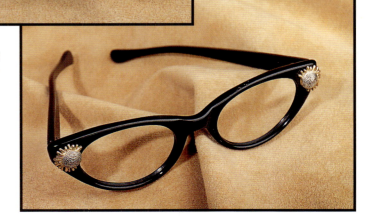

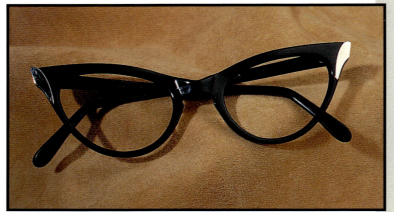

Black plastic eyewear with silver corners, marked Whitney USA. Courtesy of Barbara Blau. $30.

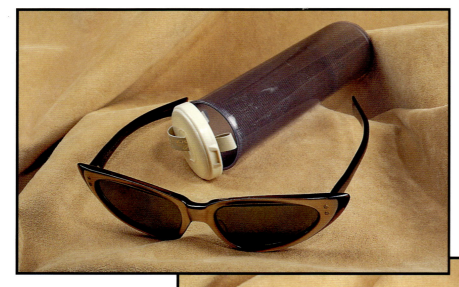

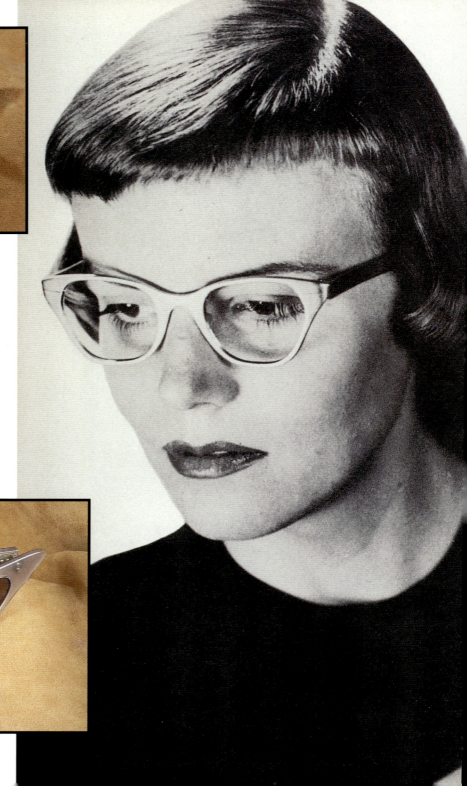

Above: Boxed pair of gray pearl plastic frames marked Sea Mist, Caloban C 86T American Optical Company, in original plastic tube and cardboard box. Courtesy of Helaine Fendelman.

Right: Light blue pearl plastic frames with elongated corners, marked Made in France. Courtesy of Helaine Fendelman.

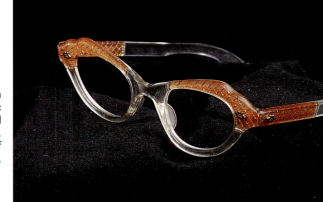

Clear and brown plaid plastic frames marked ATHWAY 346. Courtesy of Aida's Antiques.

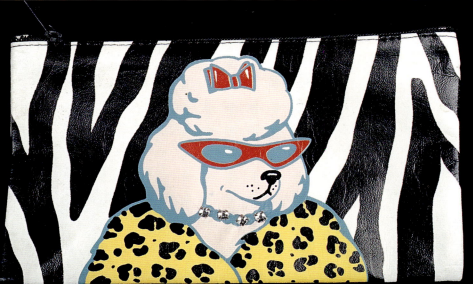

Black and white layered plastic frames for square lenses with black side pieces, marked Frame France. Courtesy of Barbara Blau. $45.

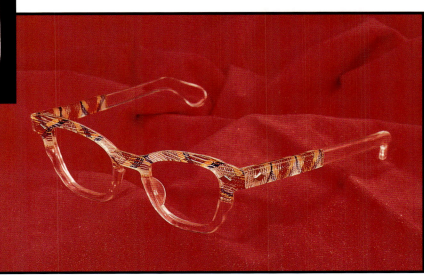

Above: Zippered pencil case with poodle in sunglasses decoration. Courtesy of Helaine Fendelman.

Right: Colorful plaid and clear plastic frames, unmarked. Courtesy of Aida's Antiques.

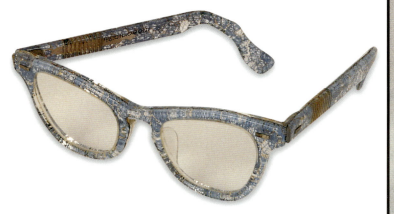
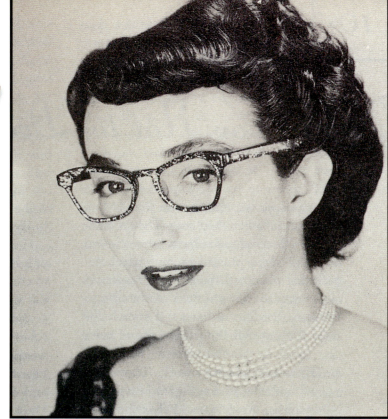
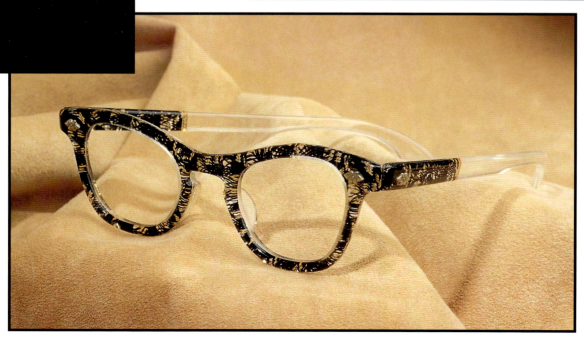

Above: Colorful plaid design on clear plastic eyewear, unmarked. Courtesy of Barbara Blau. $45.

Right: Black and gold speckled plastic frames, unmarked. Courtesy of Aida's Antiques. $20.

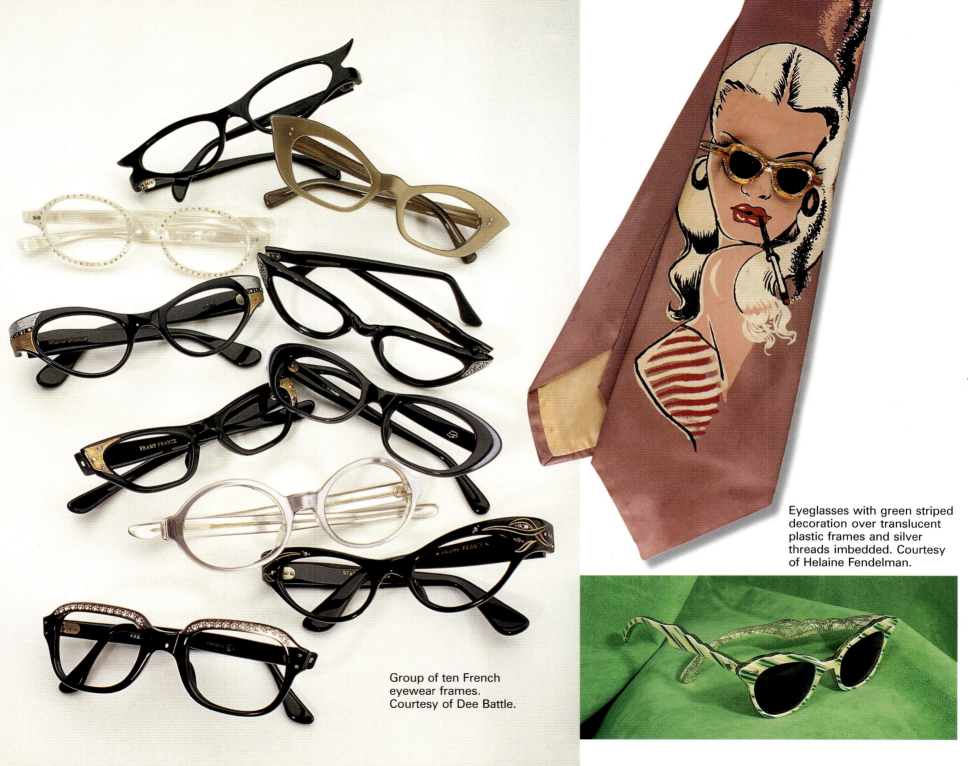

Group of ten French eyewear frames. Courtesy of Dee Battle.

Eyeglasses with green striped decoration over translucent plastic frames and silver threads imbedded. Courtesy of Helaine Fendelman.

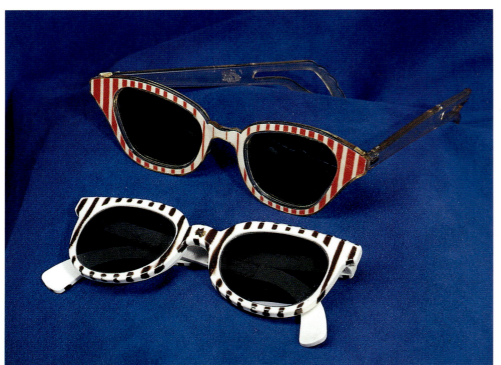

Left: Two pair of sunglasses with striped decoration. White with brown stripes marked Cool Ray Polaroid 60, clear frame with red stripes, marked Made in U.S.A. Courtesy of Helaine Fendelman.

Below: Sunglasses, Ray Ban. Metal, plastic. Bausch and Lomb, United States, c. 1950s-60s. Courtesy of The Museum of Ophthalmology, Foundation of the American Academy of Ophthalmology, San Francisco.

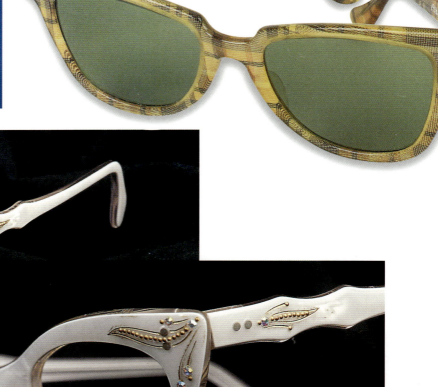

White pearl plastic frames with rhinestones marked Selecta Frame France. Courtesy of Barbara Blau. $ 25.

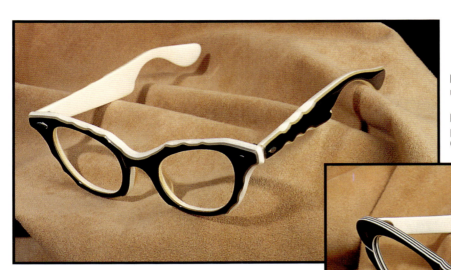

Left: Black and white layered plastic frames, unmarked. Courtesy of Aida's Antiques.

Below: Black and white shaped and layered plastic frames marked Italy and labeled "Luna Overlapped." Courtesy of Aida's Antiques.

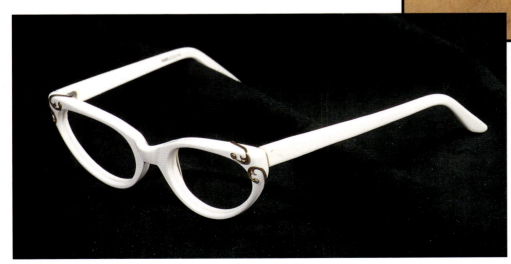

Lady's white plastic frames marked Harlequin USA 5 1/4 "See Fair." Courtesy of Barbara Blau. $35.

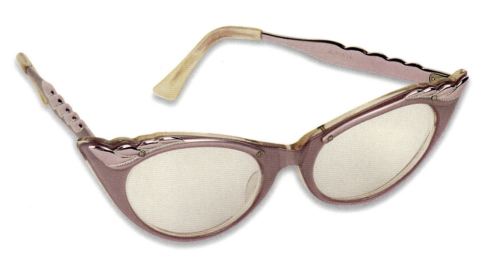

Spectacles. Plastic, metal, glass. Marked "Jason". c. 1950. Courtesy of The Museum of Ophthalmology, Foundation of the American Academy of Ophthalmology, San Francisco.

Right: White plastic frames with rhinestones in the ruffled corners, unmarked. Courtesy of Helaine Fendelman.

Below: Black frames by Raybert. Bronze eyewear with rhinestones marked USA. White eyewear with rhinestones. Courtesy of Dee Battle.

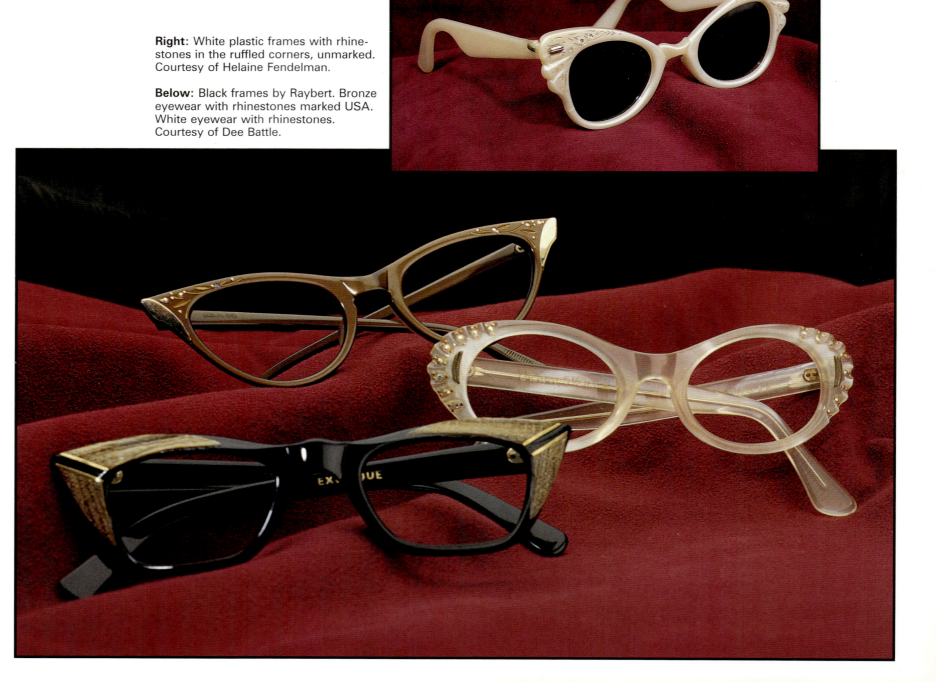

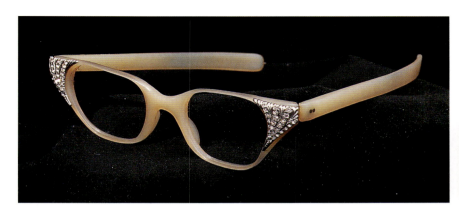

Tan Nylon frames with corner silver and rhinestone attachments and straight side pieces. Courtesy of Aida's Antiques.

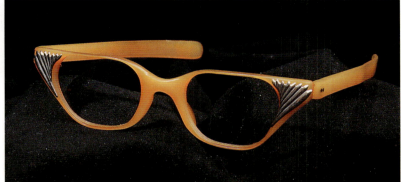

Above: Brown nylon frames with silver corner attachments, unmarked. Courtesy of Aida's Antiques. $55.

Left: Two-folding lorgnette, plastic. No lenses. France, c. 1950. Courtesy of The Museum of Ophthalmology, Foundation of the American Academy of Ophthalmology, San Francisco.

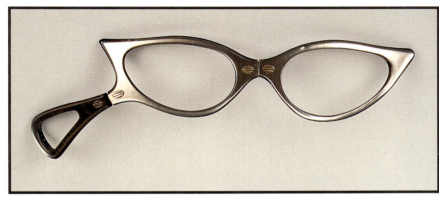

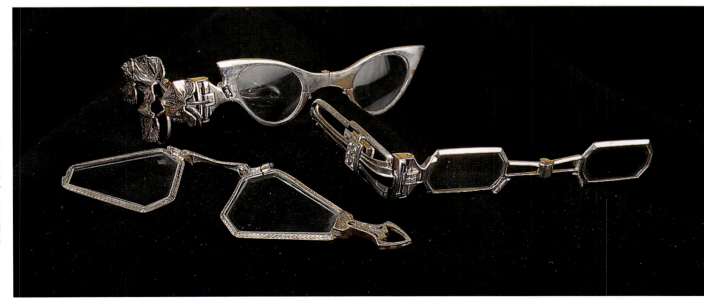

Three convertible lorgnettes, one with six-sided folding frames; one with long octagonal folding frames on a dress clip with six rhinestones and black enamel silver openwork; and a folding cat's eye silver frame with clip of four leaves marked Sterling. Courtesy of John and Valda Tull.

Right: Folding lorgnette with cream colored plastic frames decorated with gold stars, marked Made in Italy WW. Courtesy of Helaine Fendelman.

Center right: Three pair of folding lorgnettes, the gray pair marked Hong Kong, others not marked. Courtesy of John and Valda Tull.

Below: Diana Dors wearing eyewear by Oliver Goldsmith, 1959, Ass. British Corps Elstree Studio. Oliver Goldsmith Eyewear Ltd.

Bottom right: P.O.G.LTD., white frame with heart, club, diamond and spade emblems at top. Oliver Goldsmith Eyewear Ltd.

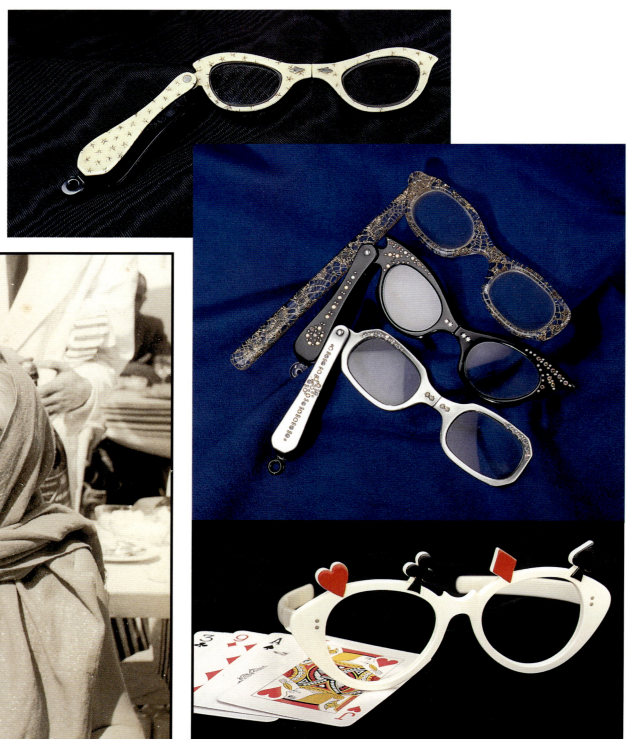

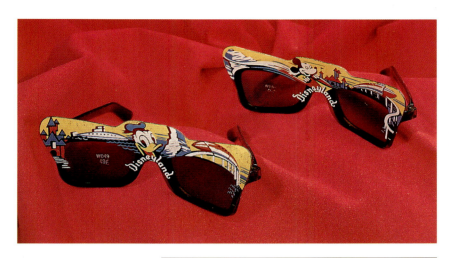

Left: Two pair of translucent plastic child's sunglasses with green shaded lenses, "Disneyland," and either Mickey Mouse or Donald Duck images painted at the tops. Courtesy of Mallory Gerber.

Below left: Display card with four pair of Tip Top child's plastic sunglasses, original price 19¢ each. Courtesy of Helaine Fendelman.

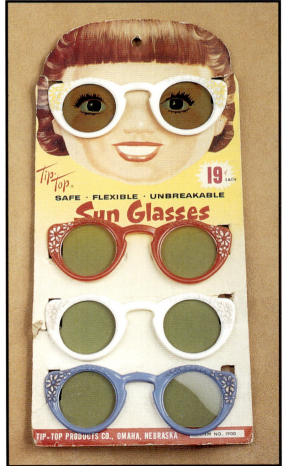

Glamour came to eyewear in the 1960s. Manufacturers created simpler, colorful sparkling styles for women and lighter weight, streamlined styles for men, in keeping with the fashions of the day. National advertising for many products included stylish people wearing sunglasses for casual activities, and the public fell into step with the trend and bought new glasses by the millions. The mail order catalogs of Sears Roebuck and Company carried magnifying eyeglasses for men and women in several styles from 1961 through 1965 at very affordable prices, $2.98 a pair.

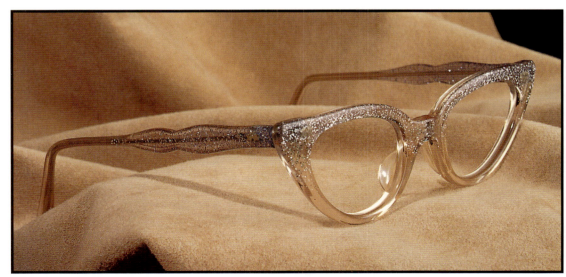

Light blue shaded translucent and silver sparkle plastic frames, unmarked. Courtesy of Aida's Antiques.

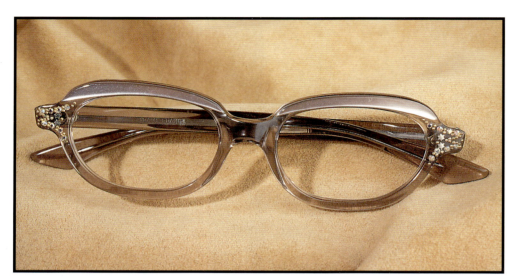

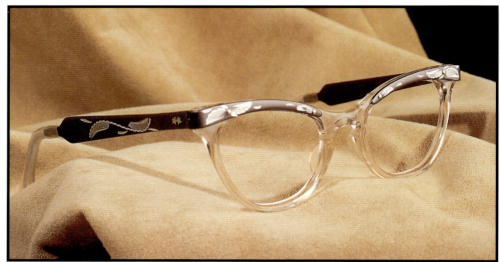

Above: Shaded translucent blue plastic frames with colored rhinestones at the corners, marked "Sharon," Frame France. Courtesy of Aida's Antiques.

Below: Black and silver aluminum eyewear over clear plastic frames marked American Optical. Courtesy of Barbara Blau. $35.

Above: Gray shaded translucent plastic and aluminum frames marked U.S.A. Courtesy of Aida's Antiques.

Below: Medium blue aluminum eyewear marked Metalite by Gaspari. Courtesy of Barbara Blau. $35.

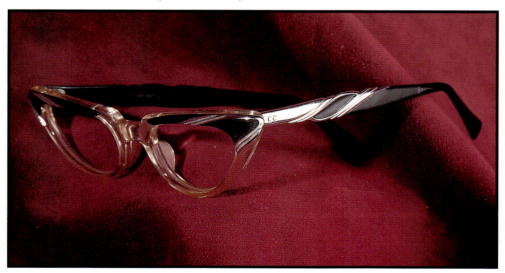

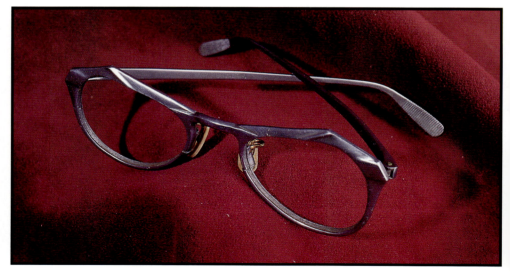

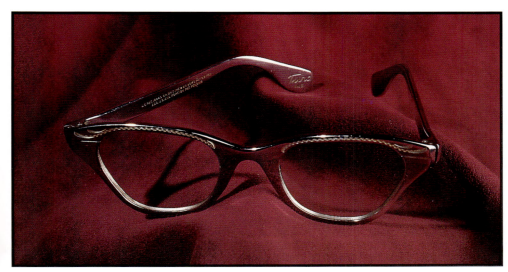
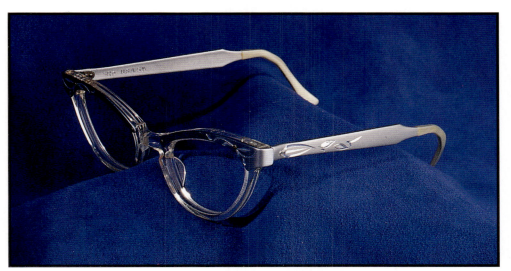

Above: Silver plastic eyewear with shaped lenses, marked Tura Inc. USA Pat 18840 and Pat. 631706. Courtesy of Barbara Blau. $35.

Below: Brown plastic frames with aluminum eyebrow trim, marked Zylite. Courtesy of Aida's Antiques. $20.

Above: Silver brushed aluminum eyewear over clear plastic frames, marked SRO USA. Courtesy of Barbara Blau. $35.

Below: Black and red layered plastic frames with gold metal corner butterfly designs and scroll decorated side pieces. Courtesy of Aida's Antiques. $20.

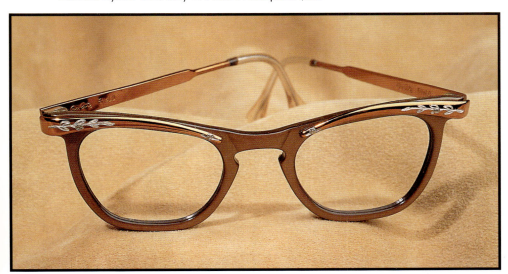
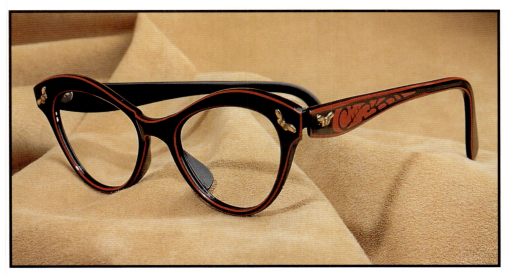

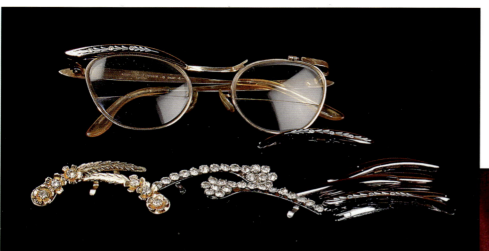

Above: American Optical 12 k gold filled with removable eyebrows. Courtesy of John and Valda Tull.

Right: Asymmetrical brown laminated plastic frames marked Frame France, Mona Lisa.
Cardboard card with plastic trims that snap on to the frames, these with pink flowers and rhinestones. Courtesy of John and Valda Tull.

Below: Brushed brown and gold aluminum eyewear marked Shuron USA. Courtesy of Barbara Blau. $35.

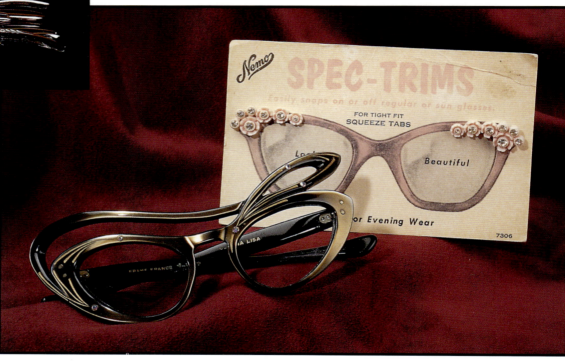

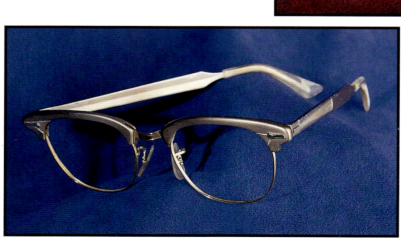

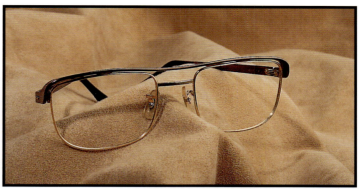

Shiny brown eyewear with gold wire frames and plastic ear pieces marked Escort Alum.<Marine> USA. Courtesy of Barbara Blau.

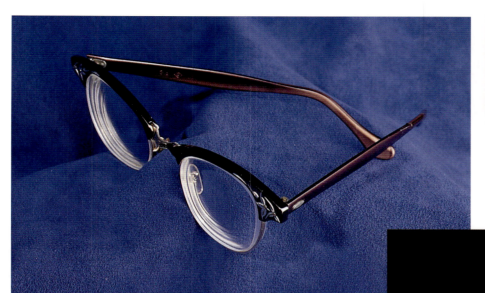

Above: Brown aluminum eyewear and gold bottom frames, marked USA. Courtesy of Barbara Blau.

Right: Two pair of 10k gold frames with gold upper frames, late 1940s to early 1950s. Courtesy of John and Valda Tull.

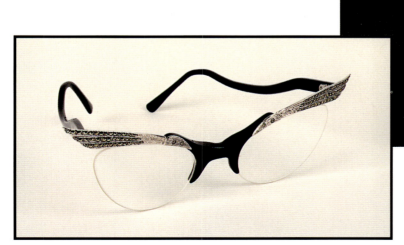

Spectacles with plastic and metal frames decorated with marcasite stones. c. 1960s. Courtesy of The Museum of Ophthalmology, Foundation of the American Academy of Ophthalmology, San Francisco.

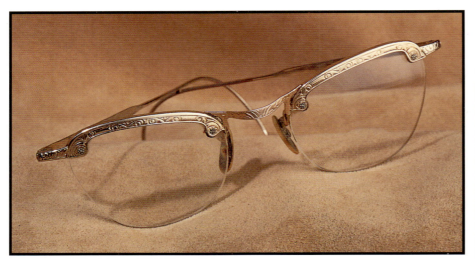

Above: Gold colored metal eyewear with curving metal earpieces, marked C.O.C. Courtesy of Barbara Blau. $35.

Right: Shaded gray translucent plastic frames with hinged and pierced side barriers, marked B=L. Safety. Courtesy of Barbara Blau. $45.

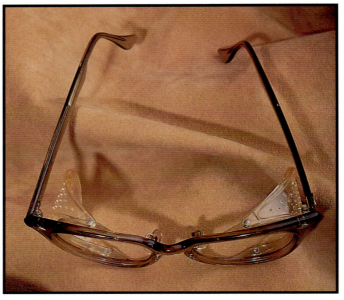

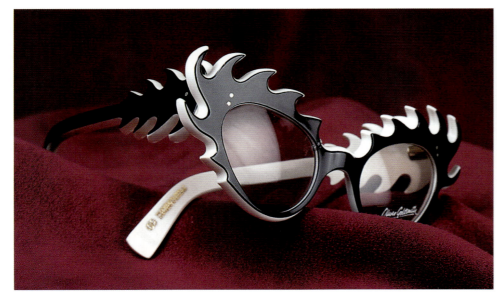

Jester, acetate, c. 1960. Oliver Goldsmith Eyewear Ltd.

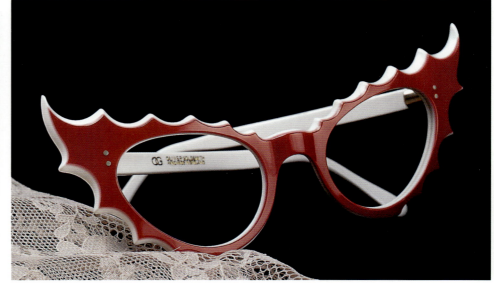

Satan, acetate, c. 1960, Oliver Goldsmith Eyewear Ltd.

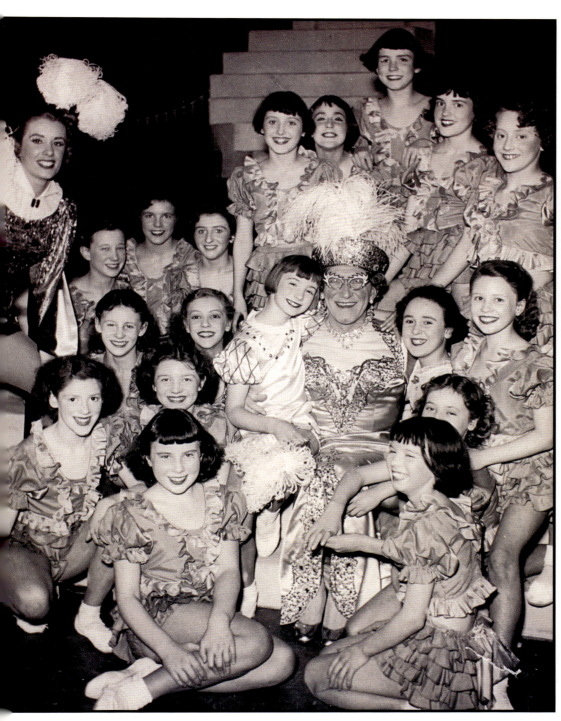

Arthur Askey wearing eyewear by Oliver Goldsmith, 1960. Oliver Goldsmith Eyewear Ltd.

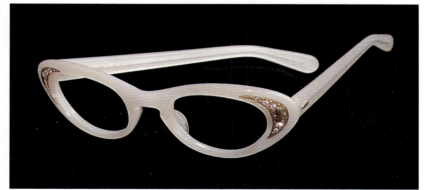

White plastic frames with rhinestones marked <Marine> Villant U.S.A. Courtesy of Barbara Blau.

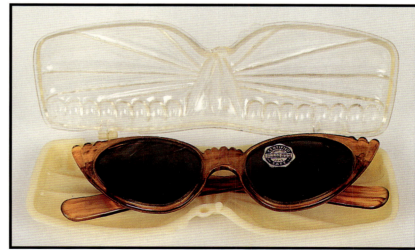

Colored lenses in faux tortoiseshell spectacles and plastic case. "Shield rite lens/Certified Sale." Case is same shape as spectacles. c. 1960. Courtesy of The Museum of Ophthalmology, Foundation of the American Academy of Ophthalmology, San Francisco.

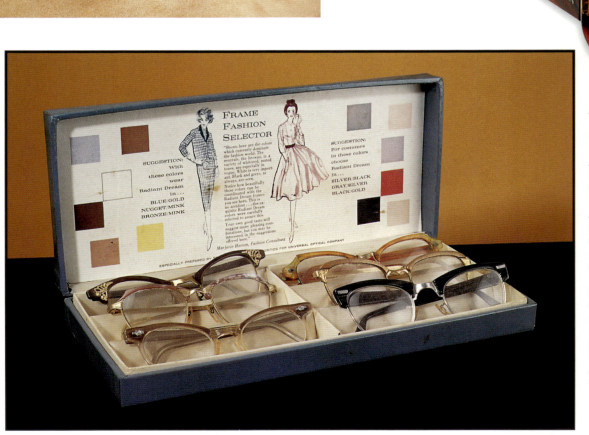

Above left: Tortoiseshell plastic thick frames marked S.R. U.S.A. 6. Courtesy of Barbara Blau. $45.

Above center: Drew, in tortoiseshell with side harps and gold brushed metal temples. Oliver Goldsmith Eyewear Ltd.

Above right: Colored spectacles, Ray-Ban. Plastic, glass. Bausch & Lomb, United States, c. 1960. Courtesy of The Museum of Ophthalmology, Foundation of the American Academy of Ophthalmology, San Francisco.

Left: Paper box display to hold six pair of glasses marked Radiant by Universal, inside lid printed "Frame Fashion Selector... Marjorie Horon, Fashion Consultant ... Especially prepared by Prominent Fashion Authorities for Universal Optical Company," containing assorted glasses from the period. c. 1960. Courtesy of John and Valda Tull.

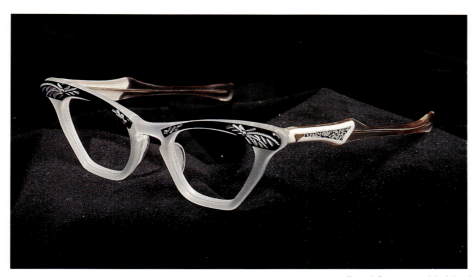
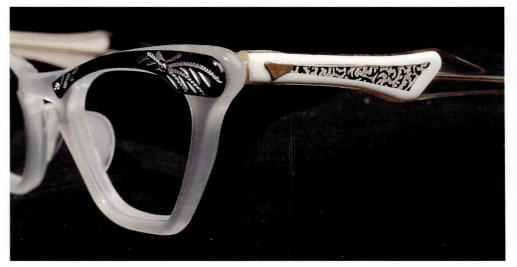

Pearl frames with black aluminum tops marked TRU-VUE 5 1/4 LO. Courtesy of Aida's Antiques.

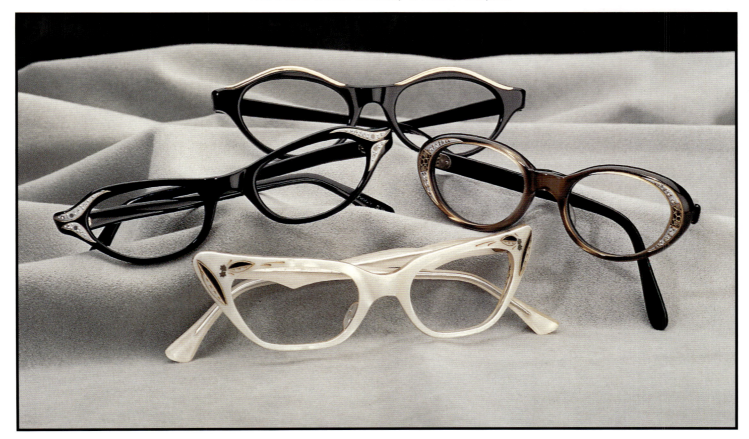

Group of four eyewear frames, unmarked. Courtesy of Dee Battle.

Right: Two Swank eyewear frames. Courtesy of Dee Battle.

Bottom left: Black, red and white layered plastic frames with scrolled corner decoration, marked Romeo 4. Courtesy of Aida's Antiques. $20.

Bottom center: Blue plastic eyewear with silver and gold side decoration, marked Shuron Alum USA. Courtesy of Barbara Blau. $25.

Bottom right: Plastic tortoiseshell frames with white accents at the top, marked Frame France. Courtesy of Barbara Blau. $30.

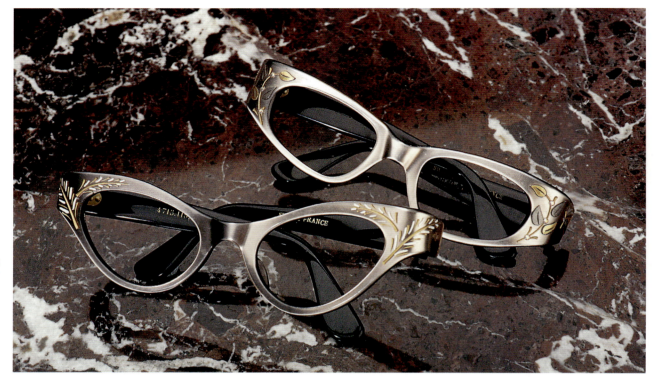

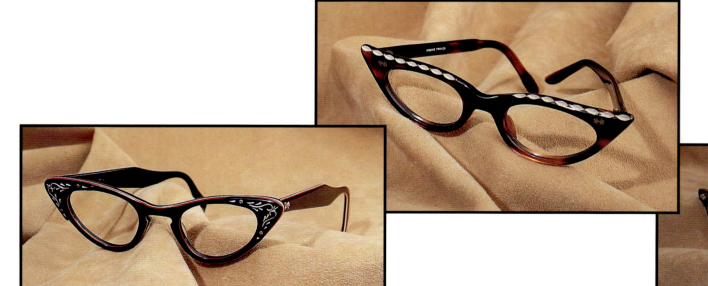

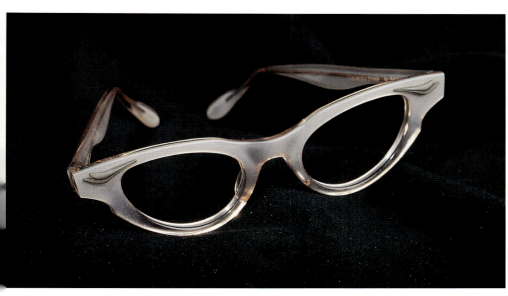

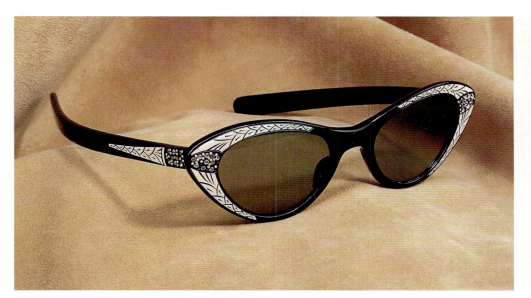

Above: Shaded clear and pearl plastic frames by Bausch & Lomb. Courtesy of Barbara Blau. $25.

Below: Child's light blue plastic frames marked S R USA 5. Courtesy of Barbara Blau. $20.

Above: Black plastic cat-eye frames with gold painted design and rhinestones in the corners, marked France. Courtesy of Helaine Fendelman.

Below: Silver and black plaid frames, unmarked. Courtesy of Aida's Antiques.

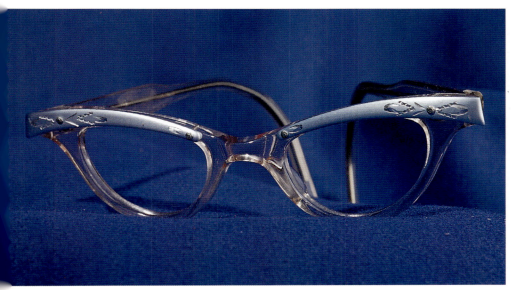

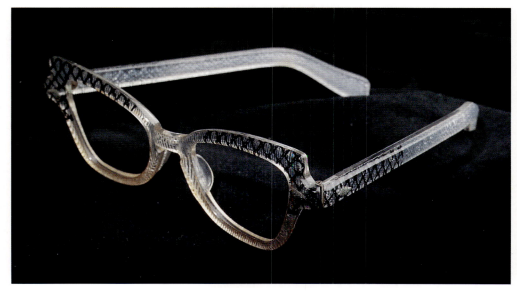

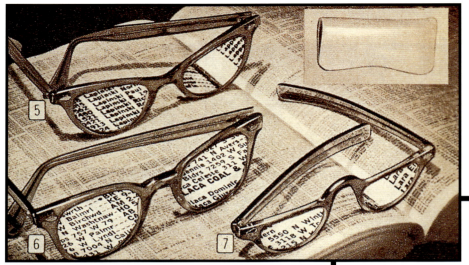
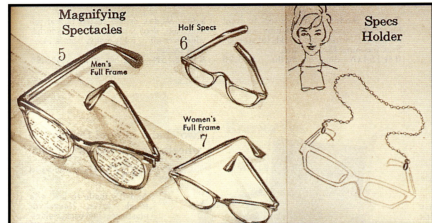
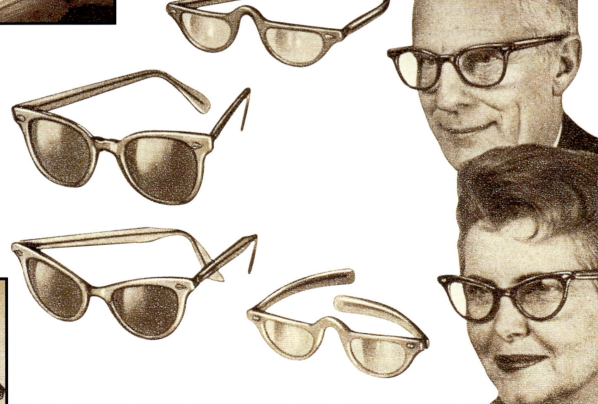
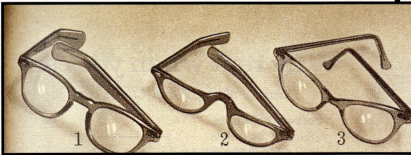

Eyeglasses available through the Sears and Roebuck mail order catalogs, 1961 through 1965.

118

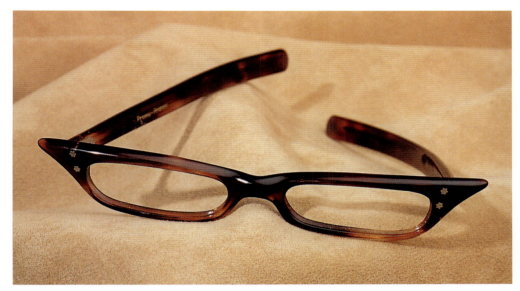

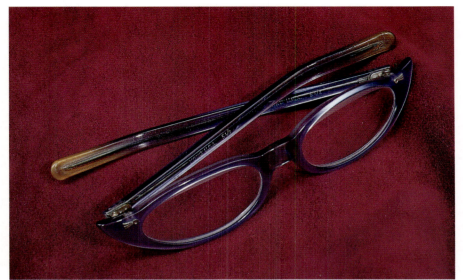

Above: Brown tortoiseshell eyewear marked Swank Opt. Frame France. Courtesy of Barbara Blau. $35.

Below: Spectacles. Plastic, rhinestones. c. 1960. Courtesy of The Museum of Ophthalmology, Foundation of the American Academy of Ophthalmology, San Francisco.

Above: Blue translucent plastic half frame reading glasses marked Kono USA. Courtesy of Helaine Fendelman.

Below: Layered half frame reading glasses with leopard spotted frames, unmarked. Courtesy of Helaine Fendelman.

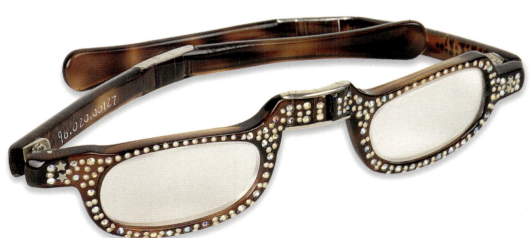

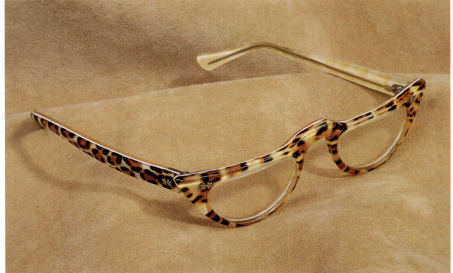

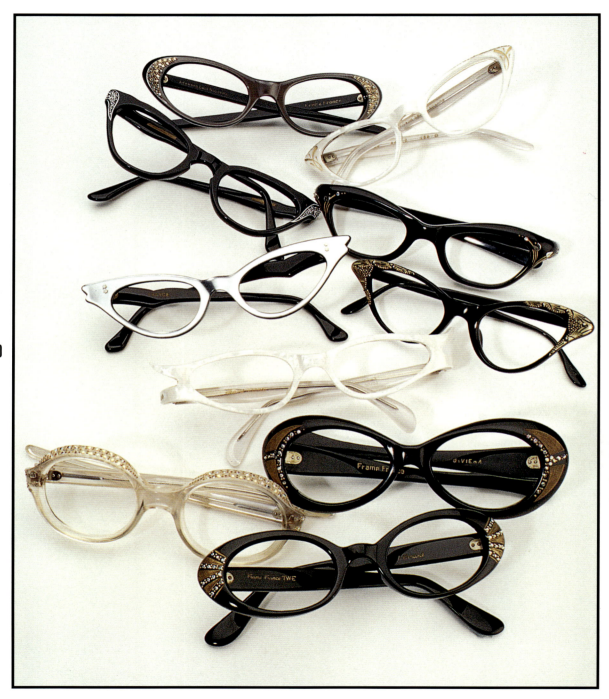

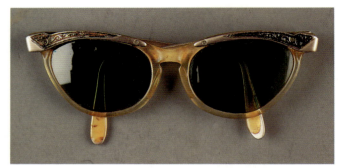

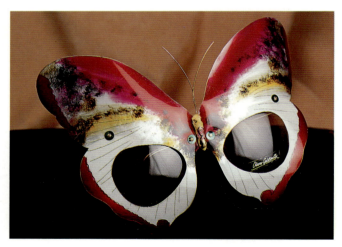

Top right: Tinted green glass in light brown plastic frames with added metal eyebrow decorations, marked Liberty U.S.A. Private collection.

Above: Butterfly, acetate with hand painted mask, c. 1962. Oliver Goldsmith Ltd.

Left: Group of ten French eyewear frames. Courtesy of Dee Battle.

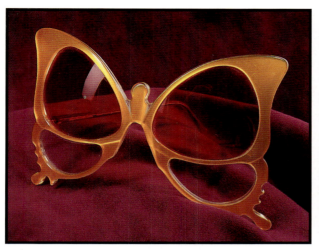
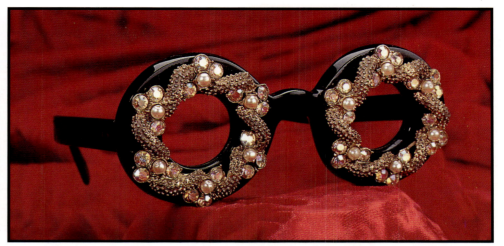
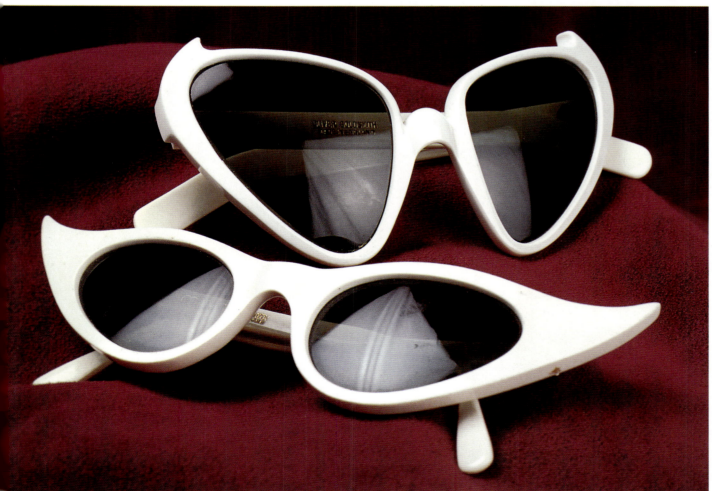

Top left: Yellow pearl plastic frames of butterfly shape with red lenses above and light pink tinted lenses below. Marked Anglo American Optical Frame England, Handmade. Courtesy of Helaine Fendelman.

Top right: Goo-Goo Decor, c. 1963, (as worn by entertainer Arthur Askey) acetate, round black frames without lenses, rhinestone and pearl with gold rope decoration. Oliver Goldsmith Eyewear Ltd.

Left: Daffy, and white cat-eye glasses. Oliver Goldsmith Eyewear Ltd.

121

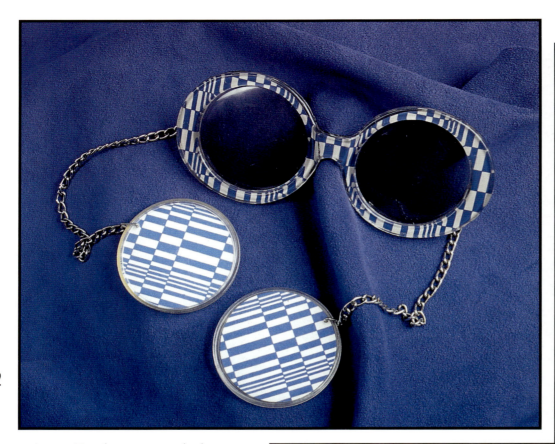

For the young and adventuresome, inexpensive sunglasses were made in exotic styles, bright colors, and unconventional parts. The temple pieces of chain with counterweights matching the frames, as shown, were funny variations of the 1960s but had counterparts in Chinese styles from centuries earlier of side strings with weights.

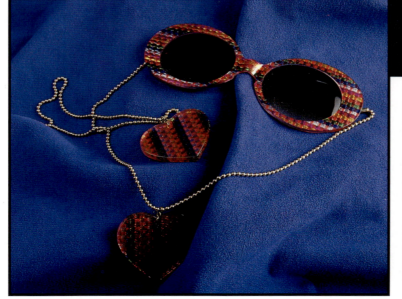

Top left: Clear plastic frames with blue and white printed pattern insets and chain ear pieces with matching plastic counterweights, unmarked. Courtesy of Helaine Fendelman.

Above: Layered plastic frames with black and white zebra stripes and chain earpieces counterweighted with matching plastic discs. Unmarked. Courtesy of Helaine Fendelman.

Left: Layered plastic frames encasing woven metallic cloth with continuous ball chain ear pieces and neck chain with matching plastic heart-shaped counterweights, unmarked. Courtesy of Helaine Fendelman.

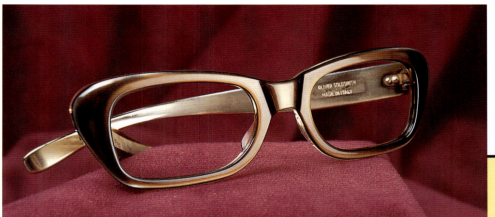

Top: Hope, acetate and metal, c. 1963, (as worn by Princess Grace of Monaco). Oliver Goldsmith Eyewear Ltd.

Center: Appo, c. 1965, (as worn by Princess Grace of Monaco) acetate and metal, tortoise frame with gold metal arms and top piece. Oliver Goldsmith Eyewear Ltd.

Bottom: Black For-her, c. 1964, with metal eyebrows and temples, Oliver Goldsmith Eyewear Ltd.

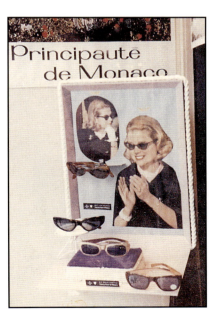

Princess Grace of Monaco wearing eyewear by Oliver Goldsmith. Oliver Goldsmith Eyewear Ltd.

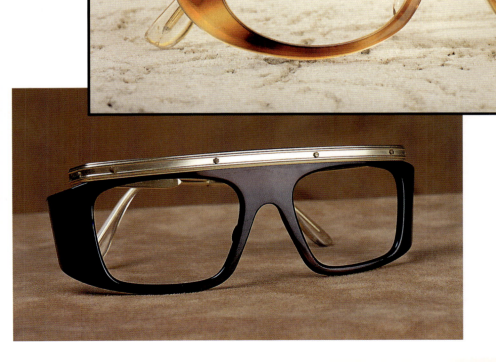

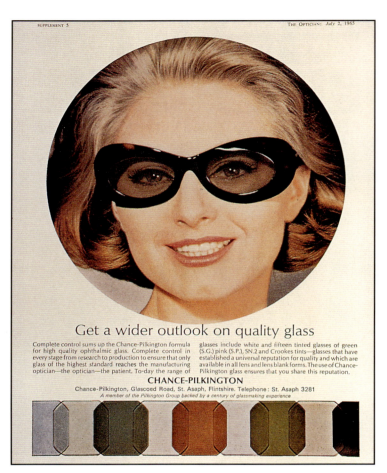

Range of tinted glass for eyewear advertised by Chance-Pilkington, 1965. Oliver Goldsmith Eyewear Ltd.

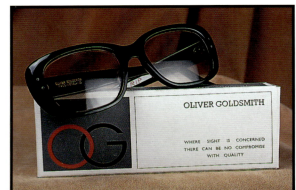

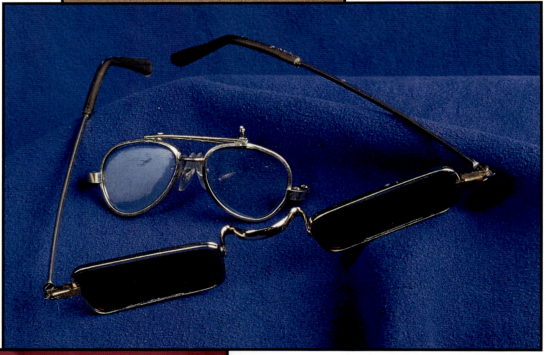

Top: "Rip," acetate, c. 1966, (as worn by Lord Snowdon) with box used in 1966. Oliver Goldsmith Eyewear Ltd.

Center: Gold tone metal frames around rose-tinted square lenses, unmarked. And a miniature pair of pilot's style sunglasses mounted as a brooch. Courtesy of Helaine Fendelman.

Left: Tortoiseshell plastic and gold metal eyewear with round lenses. Courtesy of Barbara Blau. $35.

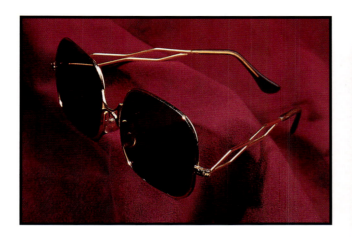

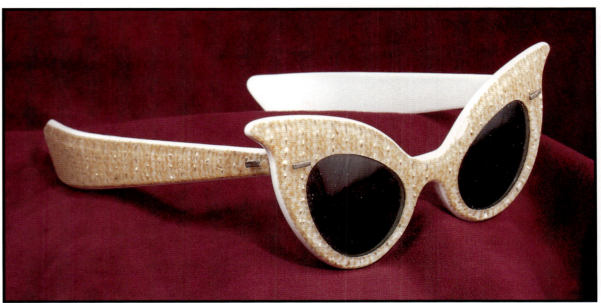

Top left: Gold metal eyewear with gray square lenses, marked Japan 529. Courtesy of Barbara Blau. $15.

Top right: Large white plastic frames with imbedded and woven metallic threads, unmarked. Courtesy of Helaine Fendelman.

Bottom left: White pearlized fancy frames with side wings, unmarked. Courtesy of Helaine Fendelman.

Bottom right: White pearlized frames with side wings ornamented with rhinestones, marked France. Courtesy of Helaine Fendelman.

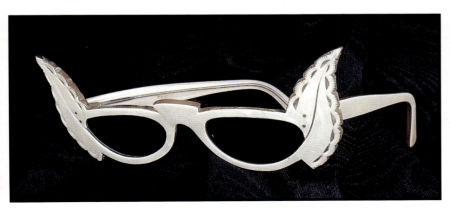

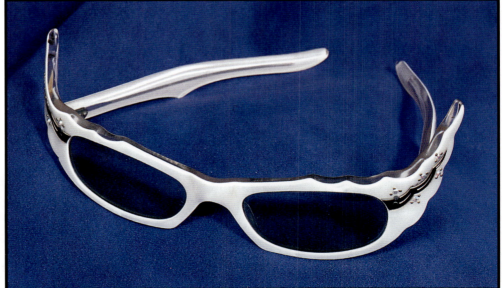

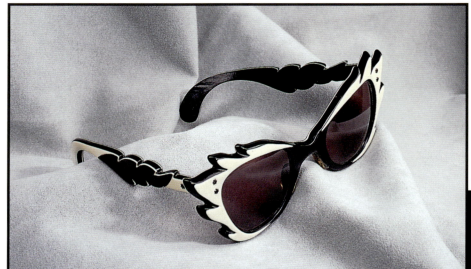

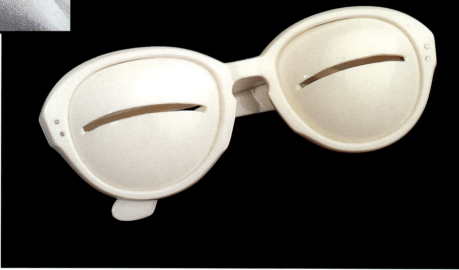

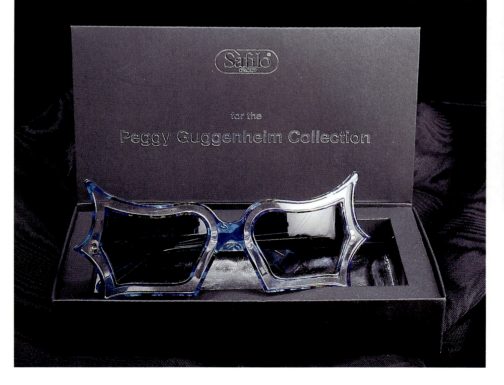

Top left: Black plastic frames with white flame edges, marked Germany. Courtesy of Helaine Fendelman.

Above: White plastic frames and lenses with open slits, from Courreges, marked France. Courtesy of Mary Ann Berlangieri.

Left: Boxed transparent layered blue plastic frames made by Sàfilo for the Peggy Guggenheim Collection, with silver protective bag. Courtesy of Helaine Fendelman.

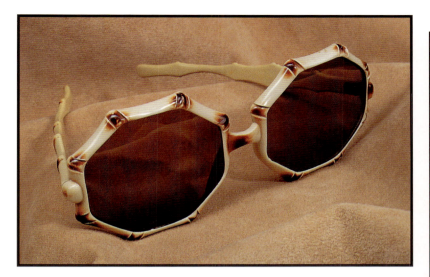

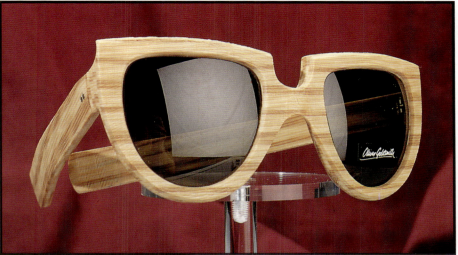

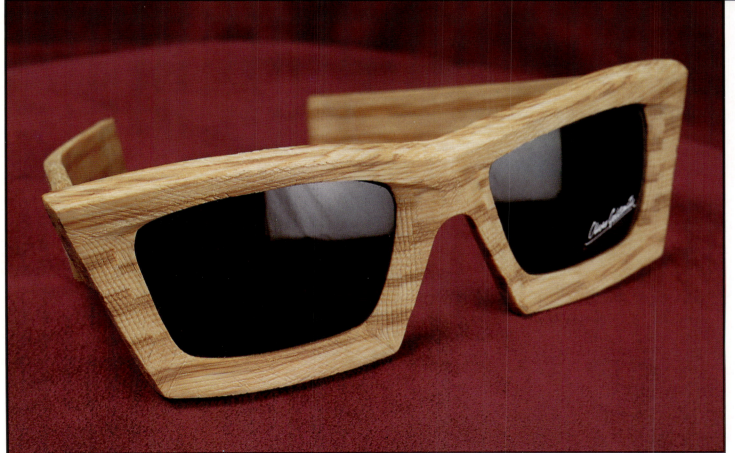

Top left: Plastic bamboo frames around octagonal lenses, marked Italy. Courtesy of Helaine Fendelman.

Top right: Y-Not, plastic resembling light brown wood grain, 1966. Oliver Goldsmith Eyewear Ltd.

Left: Bang-0n, acetate, c. 1966. Oliver Goldsmith Eyewear Ltd.

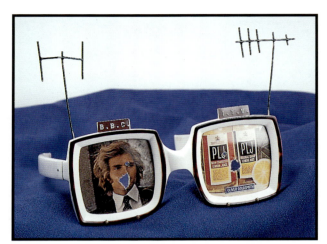

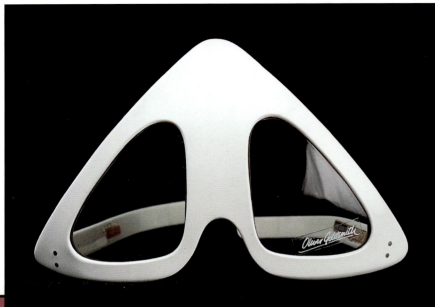

Left: "OO-er T.V. Specs," acetate, c. 1966. Oliver Goldsmith Eyewear Ltd.

Right: Pyramid, acetate, c. 1966. Made for a Vidal Sassoon hair style. Oliver Goldsmith Eyewear Ltd.

Below: "Ruanda," c. 1966, acetate, square outer frame, solid gray. Oliver Goldsmith Eyewear Ltd.

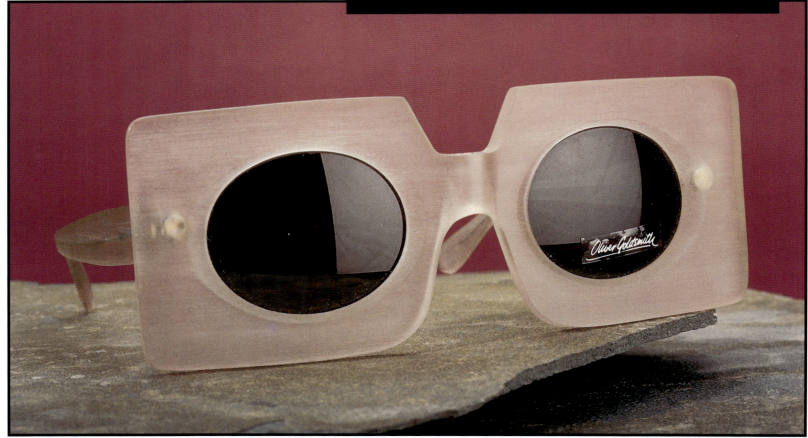

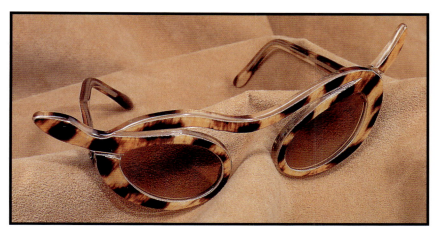

Layered plastic frames shaped as a coiled snake and marked with leopard spots, unmarked. Courtesy of Helaine Fendelman.

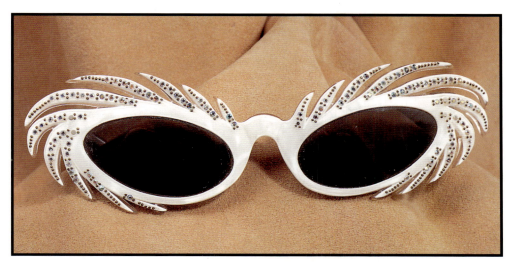

White pearlized plastic frames with feather cut edges and rhinestones, marked France. Courtesy of Helaine Fendelman.

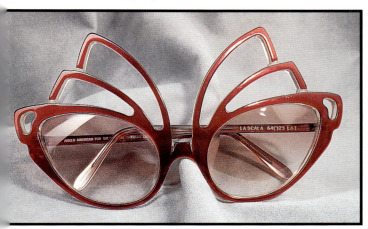

Clear and red layered frames of butterfly shape marked Anglo American For Sir Winston Frame England, LaScala 64(square)23 LA1. Courtesy of Helaine Fendelman.

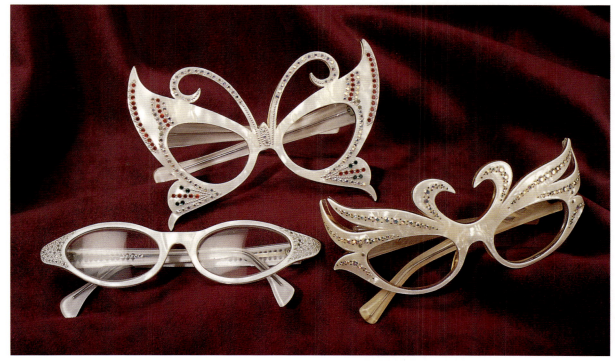

White pearl plastic frames with elaborate tops and aurora borealis rhinestones, marked Frames France. White pearl plastic frames with jeweled upper corners, marked Selecta, Frame France. White pearl plastic frames designed as a butterfly with colored rhinestones, marked ABC, Mask, France. Courtesy of John and Valda Tull.

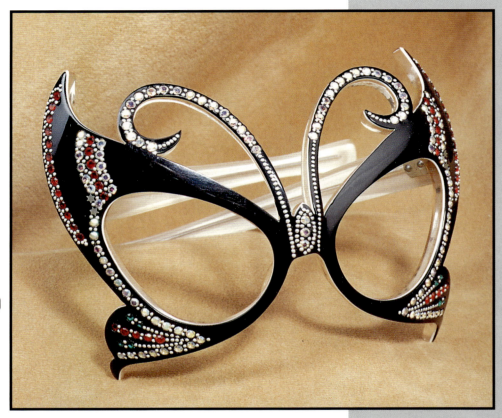
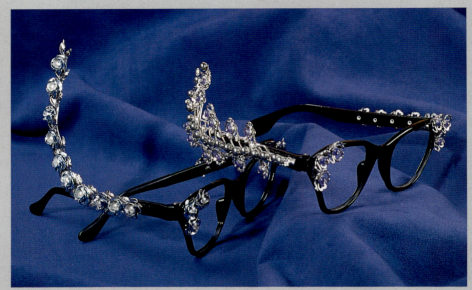
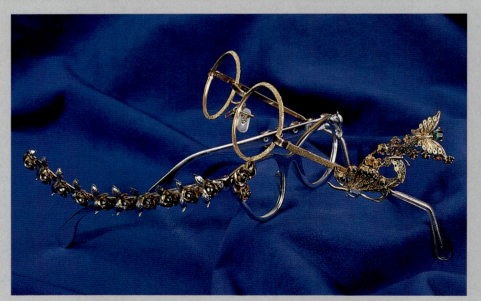

Above: Black butterfly frames design with rhinestone accents, marked France. Courtesy of Helaine Fendelman.

Two at right & opposite: Aluminum frames from Tura, late 1960s to 1970s. Courtesy of Brian K. Stewart.

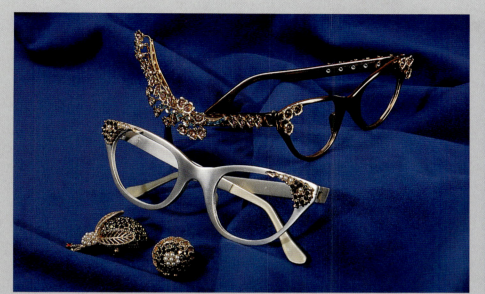
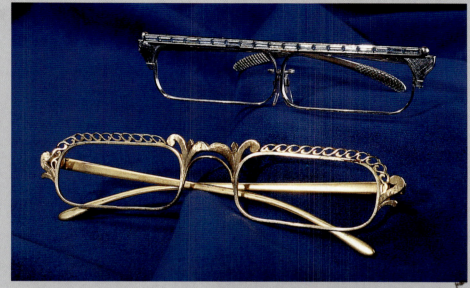
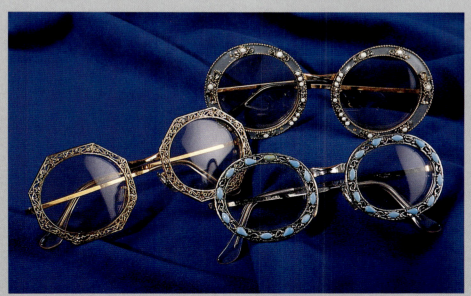
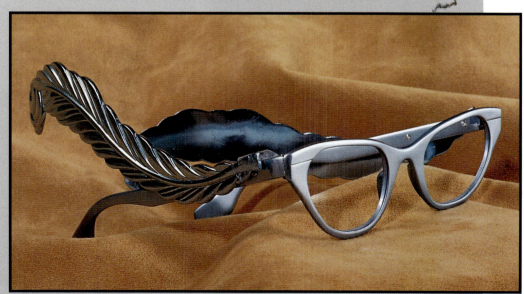

131

LATE TWENTIETH CENTURY

To associate sunglasses with glamorous individuals, Oliver Goldsmith convinced notables H.R. H. Princess Margaret, Lord Snowdon, Princess Grace of Monaco, actors Peter Sellers, Audrey Hepburn, Nancy Sinatra, Peter Lawford and Beatle John Lennon to wear his eyewear. Publicity photographs from the mid-1960s to the mid-1970s confirm his success, and added to the tendency for celebrities to hide behind dark lenses for privacy from the leering public. Fashion and jewelry designers were looking for the same glamorous associations so they teamed up with eyewear manufacturers to license their names on specific styles. Courreges, Christian Dior, and Oleg Cassini were among the first couture houses with their own lines of eyewear. Many followed suit in the following decades.

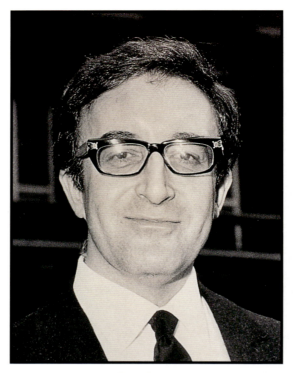

Left: Entertainer Peter Sellers wearing eyewear by Oliver Goldsmith, 1969. Oliver Goldsmith Eyewear Ltd.

Bottom left: Lord Snowdon wearing eyewear by Oliver Goldsmith, 1967. Oliver Goldsmith Eyewear Ltd.

Below: "Yu-Hu," acetate, c. 1967. Oliver Goldsmith Eyewear Ltd.

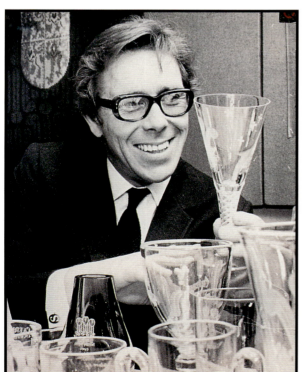

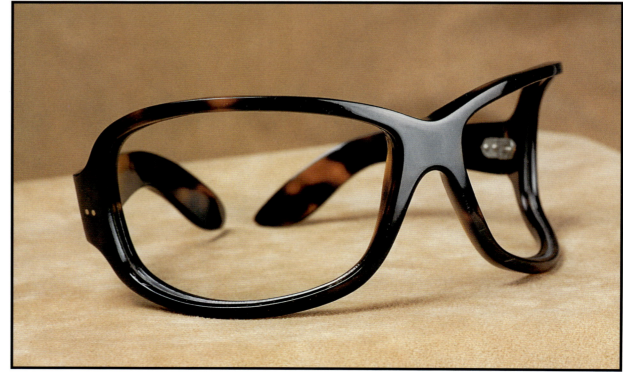

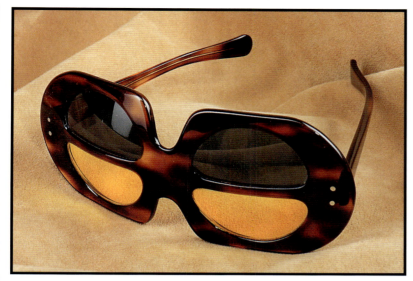

Above: Plastic tortoiseshell frames for two sets of lenses, tinted yellow and green, which can be worn upside down, marked for the retail clothing stores Peck & Peck. Courtesy of Helaine Fendelman.

Below: Two pair of Yamada sunglasses in black and tortoise. Oliver Goldsmith Eyewear Ltd.

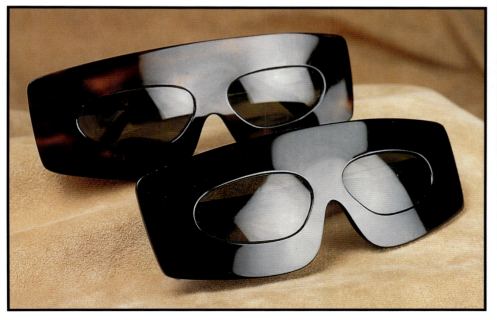

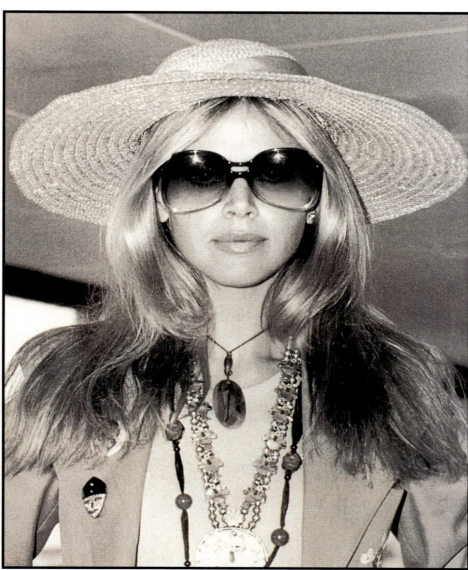

Actress Britt Ekland wearing eyewear by Oliver Goldsmith, 1968. Oliver Goldsmith Eyewear Ltd.

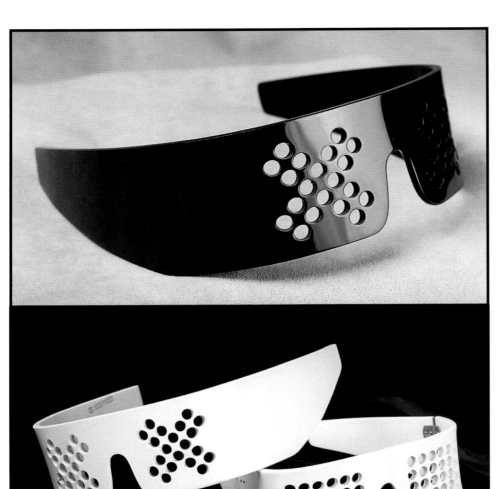

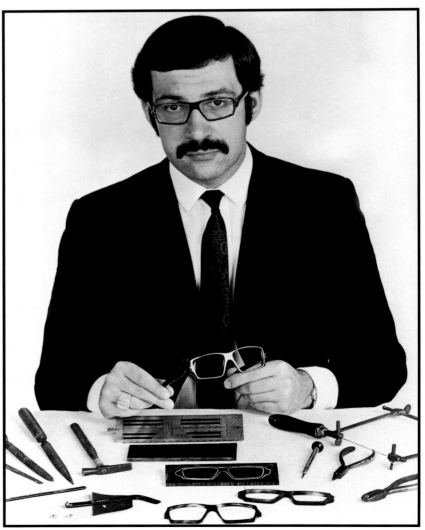

Above: Space age glasses Space Odyssey, acetate, c. 1969, in white and black. Oliver Goldsmith Eyewear Ltd.

Right: Tools and the steps used to create hand-made eyeglass frames, c. 1970. Oliver Goldsmith Eyewear Ltd.

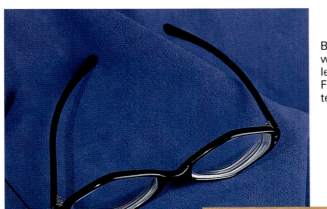

Black plastic eyewear with diamond-shaped lenses, marked Swank, Frame France. Courtesy of Barbara Blau.

Thick black plastic eyewear marked Swank, Frame, Italy. Courtesy of Barbara Blau. $35.

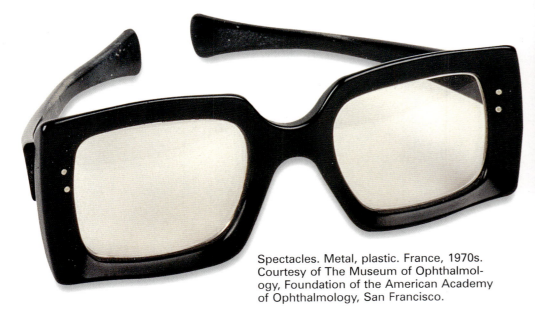

Spectacles. Metal, plastic. France, 1970s. Courtesy of The Museum of Ophthalmology, Foundation of the American Academy of Ophthalmology, San Francisco.

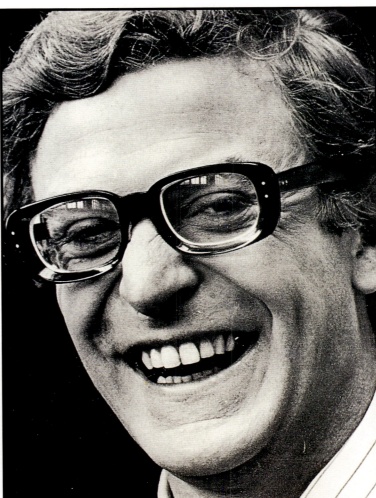

Michael Caine wearing eyewear by Oliver Goldsmith, 1970, Camera Press. Oliver Goldsmith Eyewear Ltd.

135

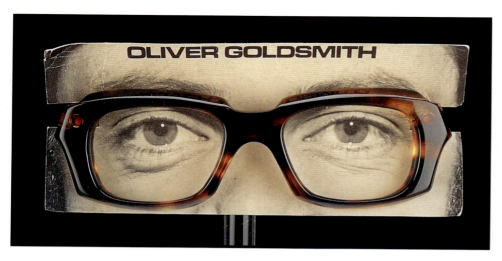
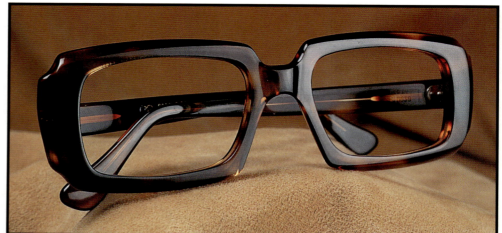
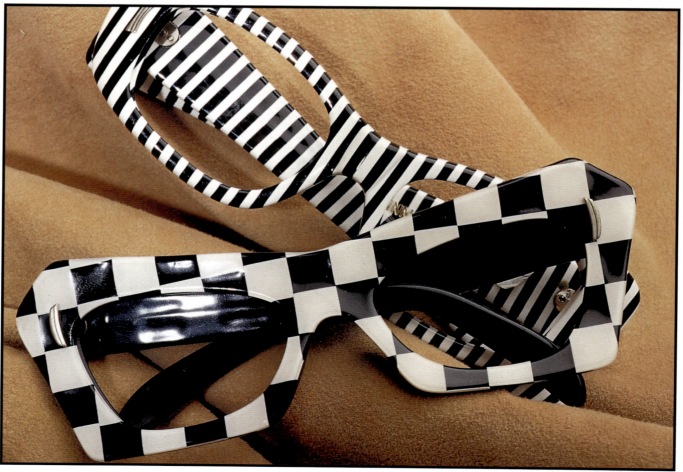

Top left: "ZAK," c. 1970, medium shell. Oliver Goldsmith Eyewear Ltd.

Top right: "Mike," c. 1975, as worn by Eric Morecambe. Oliver Goldsmith Eyewear Ltd.

Right: Black and white striped plastic frames marked "Sunmodes" SR. Black and white checkerboard plastic frames, unmarked. Courtesy of Aida's Antiques. $45 and $20.

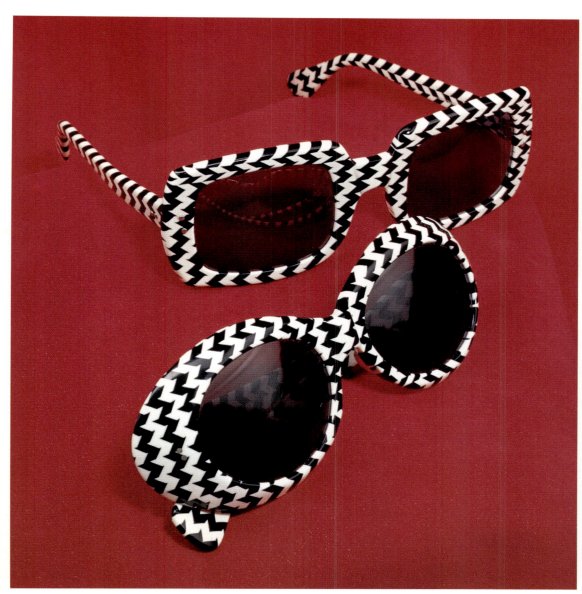

Two pair of glasses with black and white herringbone markings, one pair with oval lenses, marked A. S. Frame France. Pair with square lenses marked A Paris, Frames France. Courtesy of Helaine Fendelman.

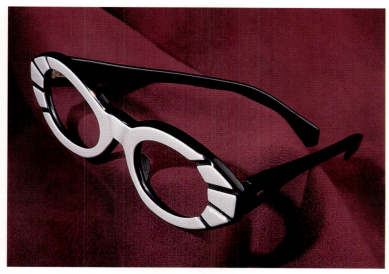

White and black eyewear marked LaLunette #1001ND. Courtesy of Barbara Blau. $45.

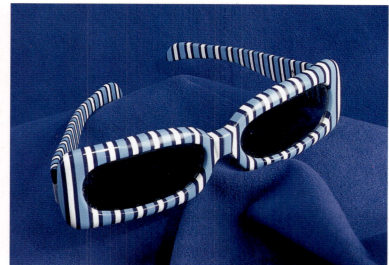

Striped plastic frames of turquoise, black and white marked Trifari, an American costume jewelry manufacturer in the mid-twentieth century. Courtesy of Helaine Fendelman.

137

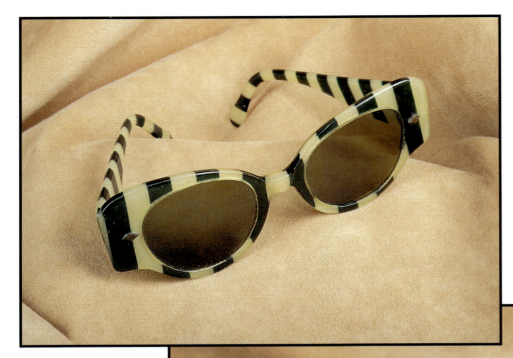

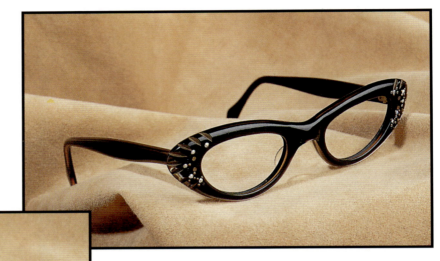

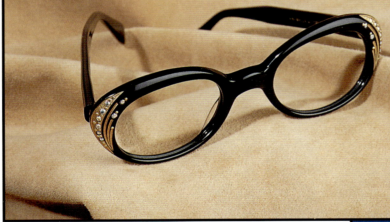

Top left: Green striped plastic frames, unmarked. Courtesy of Helaine Fendelman.

Above: Black plastic frames with corners incised and decorated, marked Kono U.S.A. Smoky, Kono Sales Co. style "Vous Gogo." Courtesy of Aida's Antiques.

Left: Black plastic frames with gold incised and rhinestone decorated corners, marked Frame made in Germany, ">Sibylle< 135 schw." Courtesy of Aida's Antiques.

Child's light blue aluminum and clear plastic frames marked "USA." Courtesy of Barbara Blau. $20.

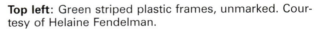

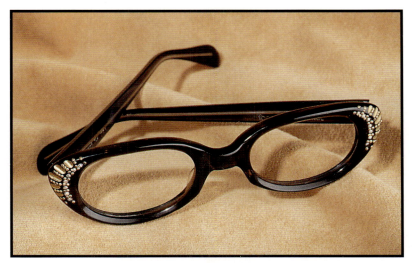

Brown translucent plastic frames with rhinestone corners, marked Foremost U.S.A. Courtesy of Aida's Antiques.

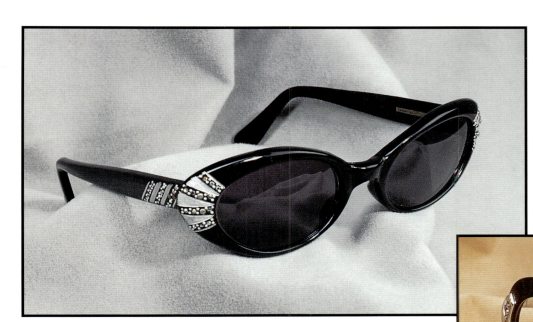

Black frames with silver paint and rhinestones at the corners, marked Qualite France, Frame France TWEC. Courtesy of Helaine Fendelman.

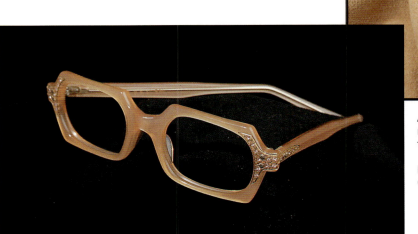

Above: Black plastic frames with purple rhinestones and silver arms, unmarked. Courtesy of Aida's Antiques.

Left: Pink plastic eyewear with rhinestones by Comet USA. Courtesy of Barbara Blau. $35.

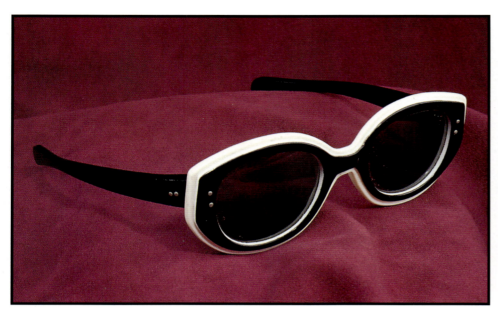

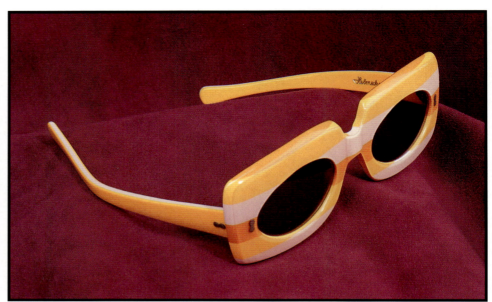

Above: Black and white plastic frames marked France. Courtesy of Helaine Fendelman.

Below: Dark brown plastic frames marked Flair Originals Frame Italy "FlairNike." Courtesy of Barbara Blau. $45.

Above: Orange plastic frames with striped pattern, marked Helmecke. Courtesy of Helaine Fendelman.

Below: Translucent clear plastic frames with silver and turquoise metallic lines imbedded, unmarked. Courtesy of Helaine Fendelman.

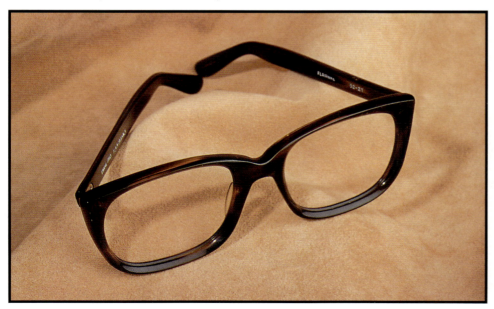

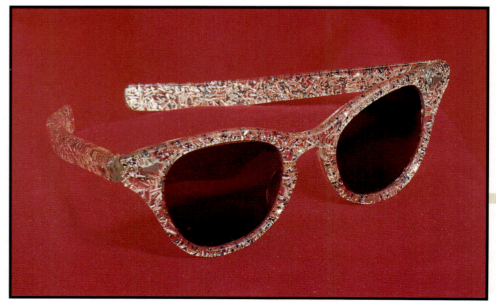

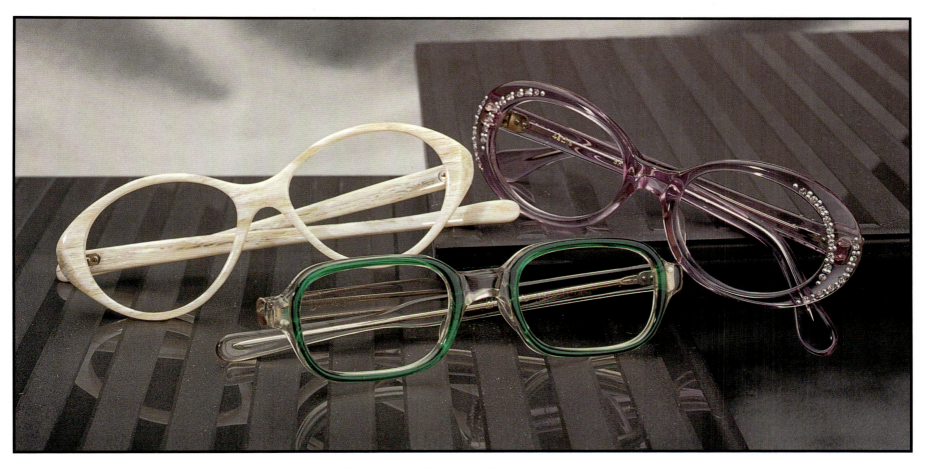

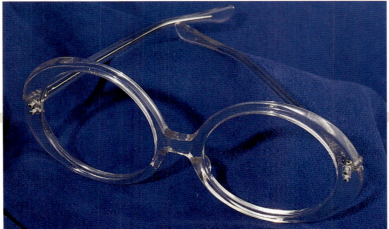

Above: Green eyewear frames by BelAir. Tan woodgrain eyewear by Zyloware. Purple eyewear by Sandra Deluxe. Courtesy of Dee Battle.

Left: Clear plastic eyewear with large round lenses, marked HOE USA. Courtesy of Barbara Blau. $35.

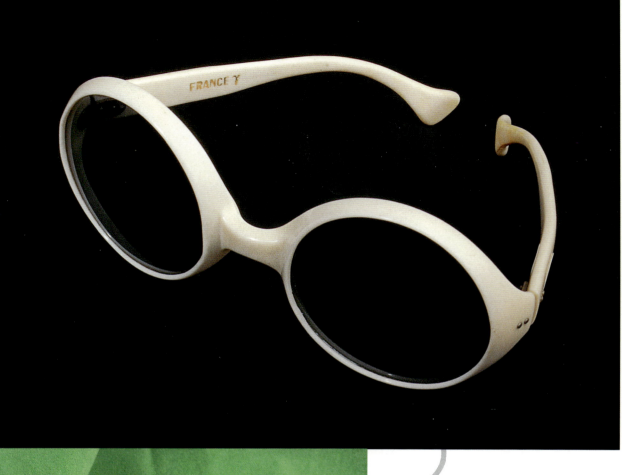

Large white plastic frames with tinted round lens, marked France. Courtesy of Barbara Blau. $15.

Red frames with imbedded woven cane straw, marked Anne Marie Perris, Frame Italy 7600, 158 P. Courtesy of Helaine Fendelman.

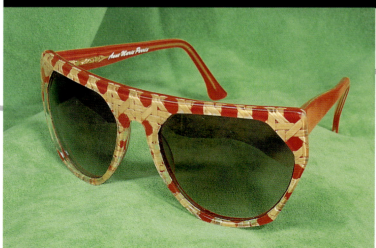

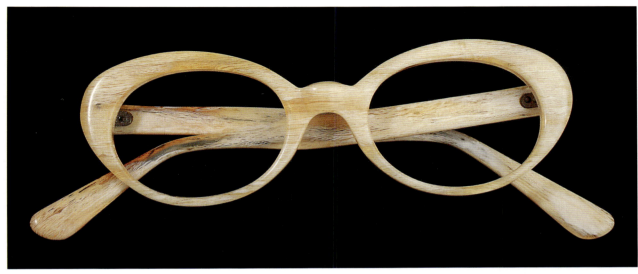 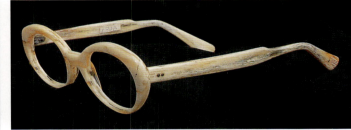

Wood grain plastic frames for oval lenses, marked U.S.A. Courtesy of Barbara Blau. $25.

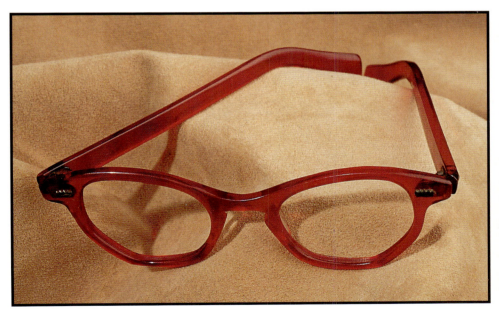

Red plastic eyewear, unmarked. Courtesy of Barbara Blau. $30.

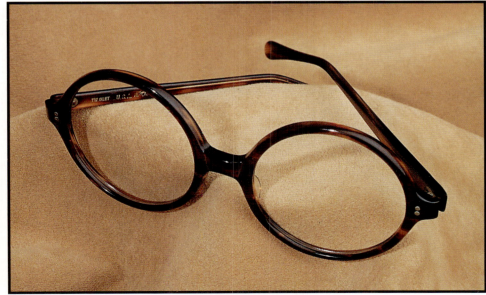

Brown tortoiseshell plastic eyewear marked TW GLET USA R.O.C. Courtesy of Barbara Blau. $35.

Right: Yellow plastic frames painted with green and purple geometric design, unmarked. Courtesy of Helaine Fendelman.

Below: Yellow patterned plastic eyewear with brown and white geometric design, marked B&L Rayban USA "Tamarin." Courtesy of Barbara Blau. $75.

Lower right: Mottled green slag marked Made in Italy. Courtesy of Helaine Fendelman.

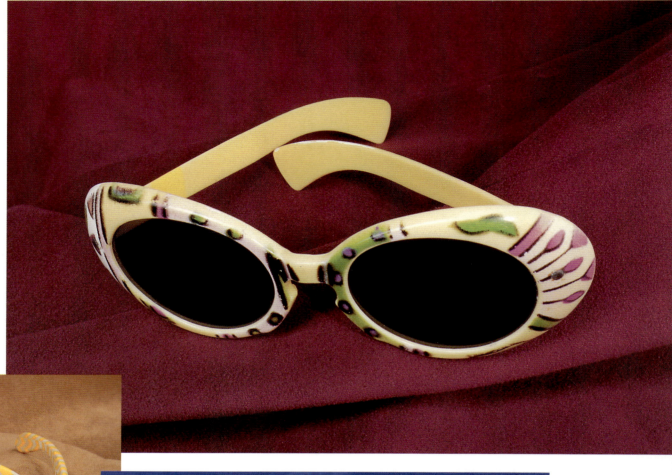

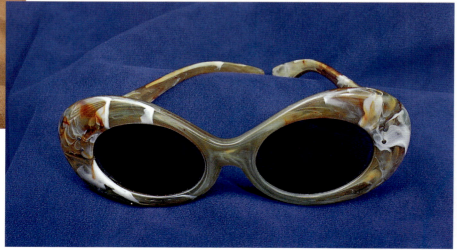

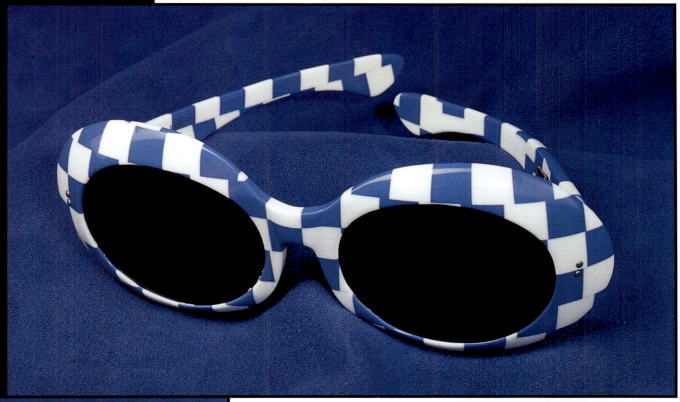

Blue and white squares, paper label reads: Designed by Emilie Roberts style 5722   5.00. Arm marked France. Courtesy of Helaine Fendelman.

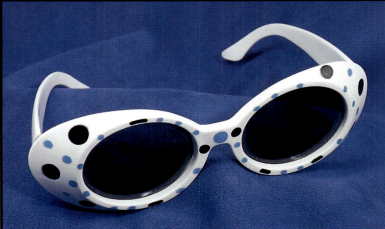

White plastic with painted black and blue dots, arms marked F G USA. Courtesy of Helaine Fendelman.

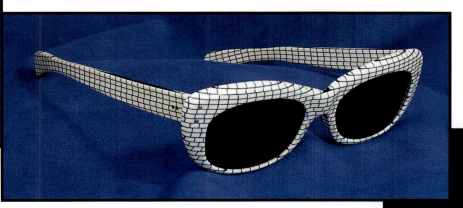

White frames with black brick pattern, unmarked. Courtesy of Helaine Fendelman.

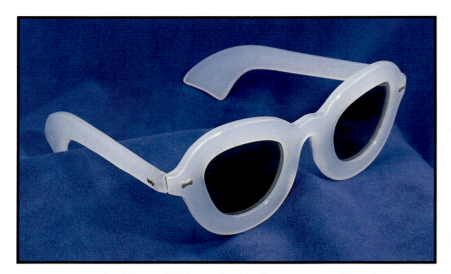

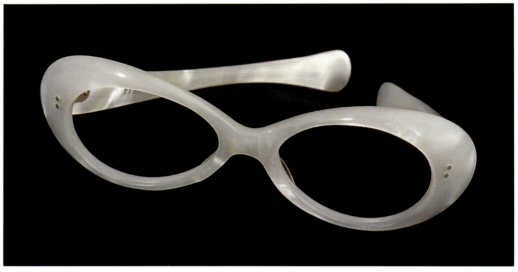

Above: Thick pearl white frames, unmarked. Courtesy of Helaine Fendelman.

Right: Lady's white mother-of-pearl plastic frames marked Frame France. Courtesy of Barbara Blau. $35.

Below: Ogle, in bright red. Oliver Goldsmith Eyewear Ltd.

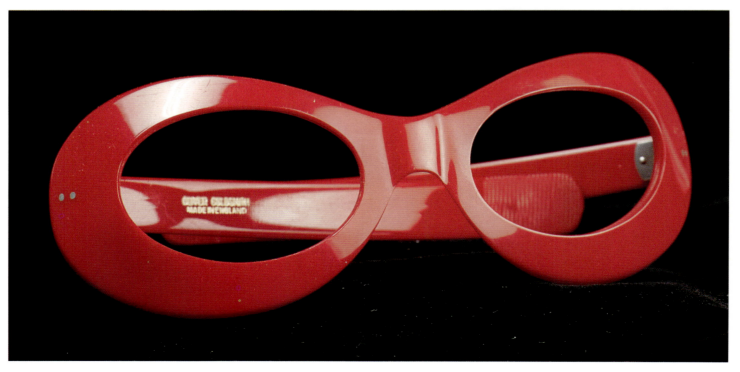

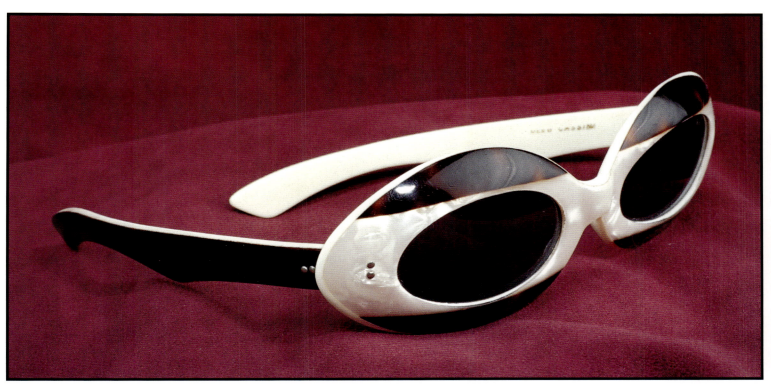

Left: Oval plastic tortoiseshell and pearl frames marked for clothing designer Oleg Cassini, France. Courtesy of Helaine Fendelman.

Bottom left: White pearlized plastic frames with wedge-shaped lenses, marked Made in France. Courtesy of Helaine Fendelman.

Bottom right: Cream colored hard plastic with black diagonal lines, unmarked. Courtesy of Helaine Fendelman.

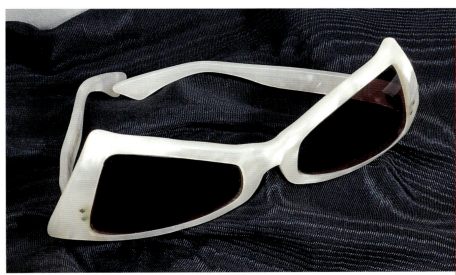

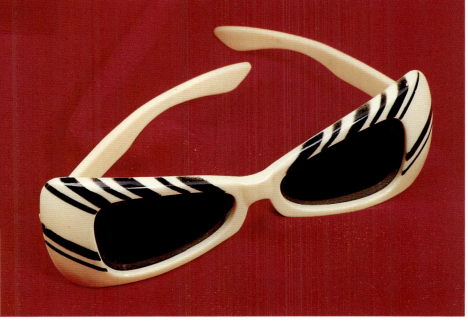

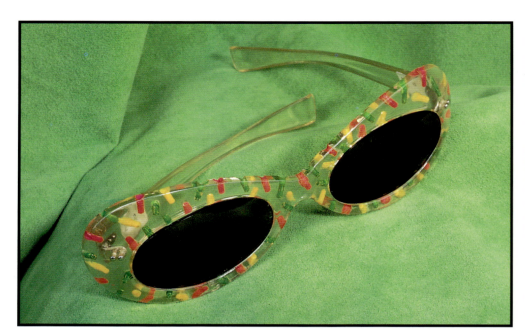

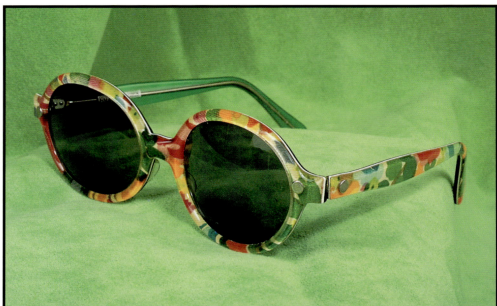

Above: Clear plastic with imbedded yellow, green, and red drilled holes, paper label reads 241 B. Courtesy of Helaine Fendelman.

Below: Orange da-glo translucent frames, unmarked. Courtesy of Helaine Fendelman.

Above: Colorful and bright green layered plastic frames, marked Lumar U.S.A. Courtesy of Helaine Fendelman.

Below: Pink and white layered frames, white arms marked Reynaud USA. Courtesy of Helaine Fendelman.

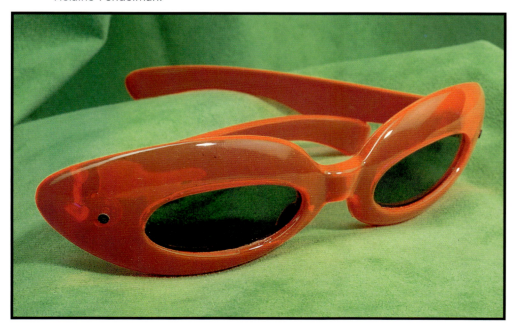

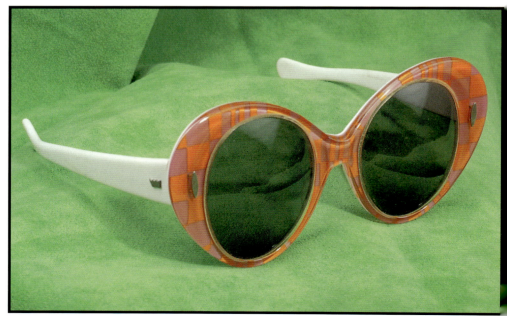

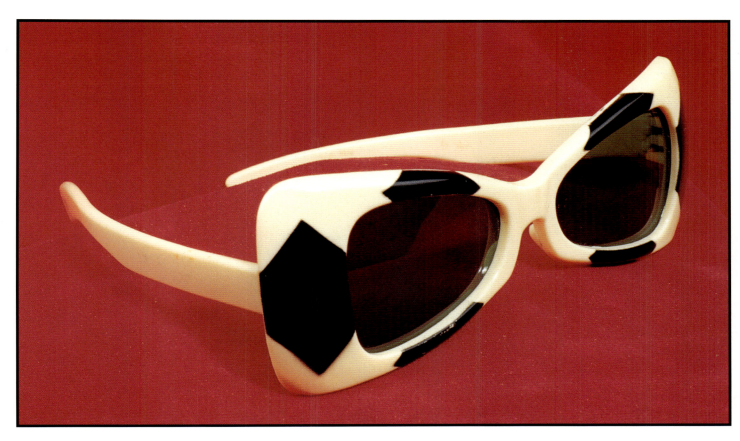

Left: Cream colored frames with black painted diamonds, unmarked. Courtesy of Helaine Fendelman.

Bottom left: Molded plastic with two snakes and slats, no lenses, marked Taiwan. Courtesy of Helaine Fendelman.

Below: White frames with black line frame. Oliver Goldsmith Eyewear Ltd.

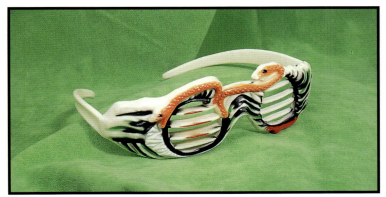

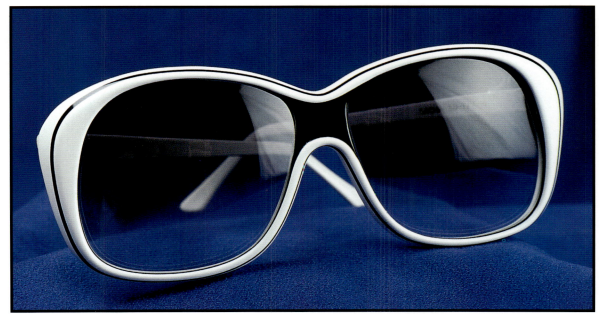

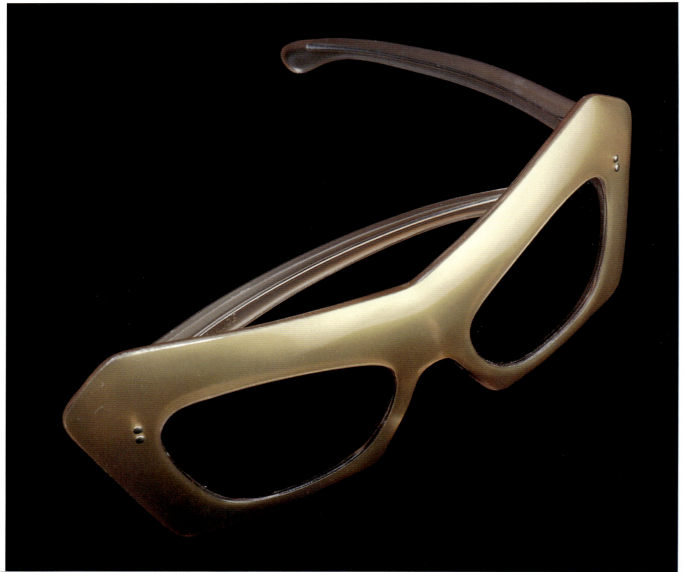

Top: Gold pearl plastic deep frames, marked France. Courtesy of Helaine Fendelman.

Bottom: Orange plastic frames marked "L. Evard," Frame France TWEC. Courtesy of Aida's Antiques.

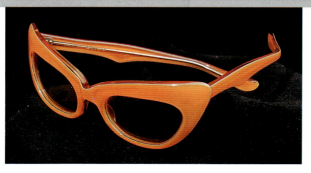

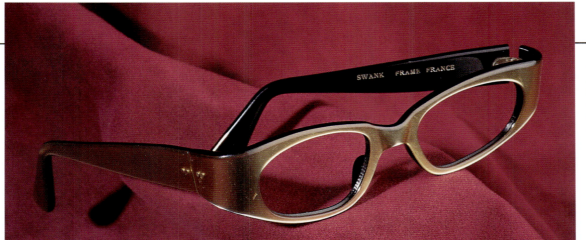

Gold plastic eyewear with black inside surface, marked Swank Frame France. Courtesy of Barbara Blau. $45.

Eyeglass manufacturers Swank of France, Safilo of Italy, and Tura of the United States and others grew large making new eyeglass and sunglasses designs for fashion houses to show with their runway collections and sell in international boutiques.

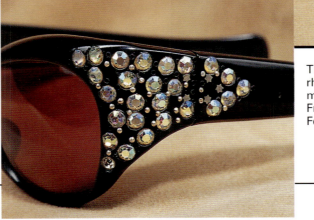

Thick black frames with rhinestones in the corners, marked Swank Opt. Frames France. Courtesy of Helaine Fendelman.

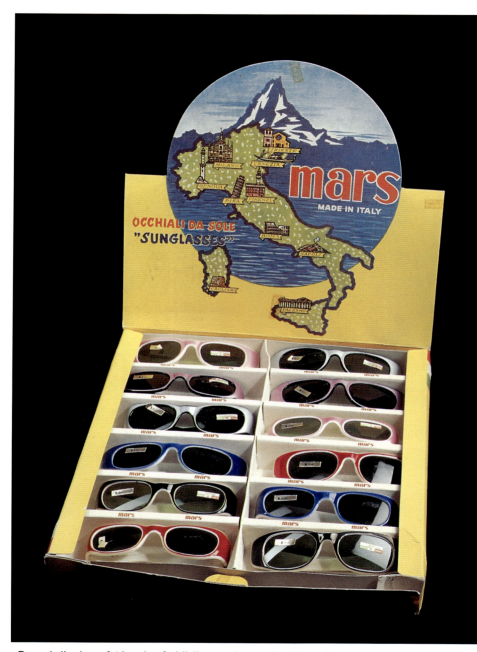

Boxed display of 12 pair of child's sunglasses by Mars, Milano, Italy, styles Capri and Dixie, original price $1 each. Courtesy of Helaine Fendelman.

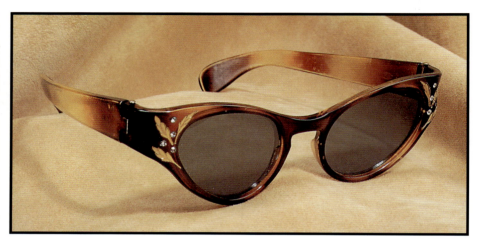

Plastic tortoiseshell cat eye frames with corner decorations of gold leaves and rhinestones, marked FG USA. Courtesy of Helaine Fendelman.

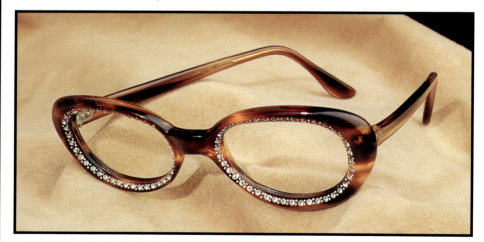

Brown tortoiseshell plastic frames with rhinestones around the lenses, marked Frame Italy. Courtesy of Aida's Antiques.

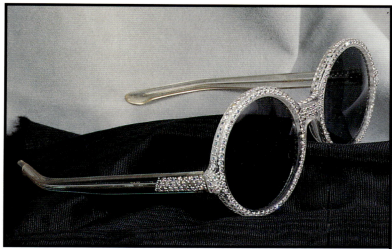

Clear plastic frames with rhinestones around round lenses, marked L. Evrard, Frame France TWE. Courtesy of Helaine Fendelman.

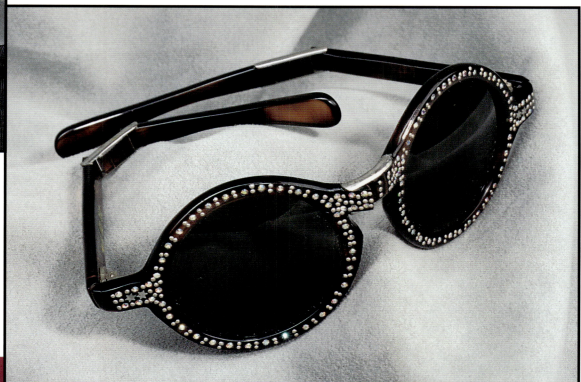

Above: Folding plastic tortoiseshell frames with rhinestone decoration around the lenses, marked Allan Optical, Frames Hong Kong. These fold into a tight circle the size of one lens. Courtesy of Helaine Fendelman.

Left: Tortoiseshell plastic eyewear with rhinestones and green lenses, marked May USA. Courtesy of Barbara Blau. $35.

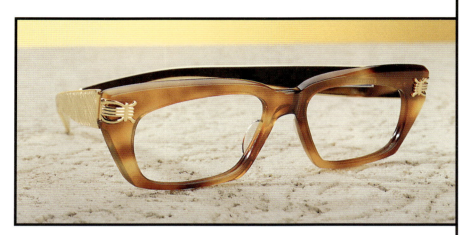

"Clent Goldside," c. 1974, (as worn by Peter Sellers) tortoise frame with gold brushed arms. Oliver Goldsmith Eyewear Ltd.

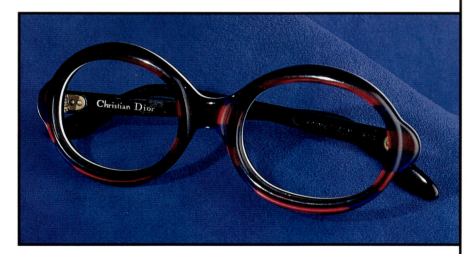

Layered plastic eyewear with red and blue horizontal striped plastic lenses and ear pieces, marked for clothing designer Christian Dior, Frame Italy. Courtesy of Barbara Blau. $75.

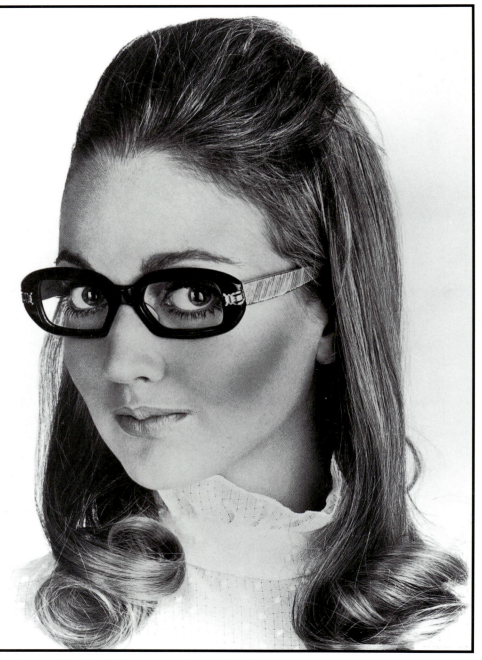

Eyeglasses with plastic frames, c. 1975, and gold metal temples. Oliver Goldsmith Eyewear Ltd.

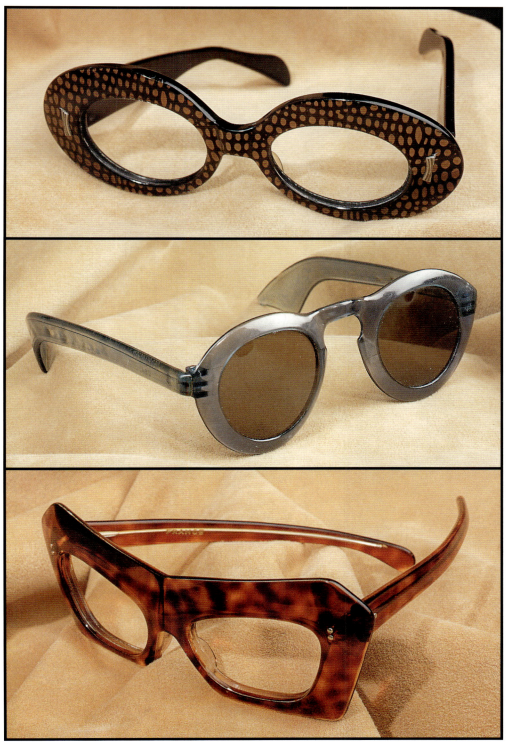

Top: Thick black plastic frames with copper chips marked Sunmodes SR. Courtesy of Aida's Antiques.

Center: Green plastic frames marked Des. Pat. 114260 U.S.A. Courtesy of Helaine Fendelman.

Bottom: Thick tortoiseshell plastic frames marked France. Courtesy of Aida's Antiques. $45.

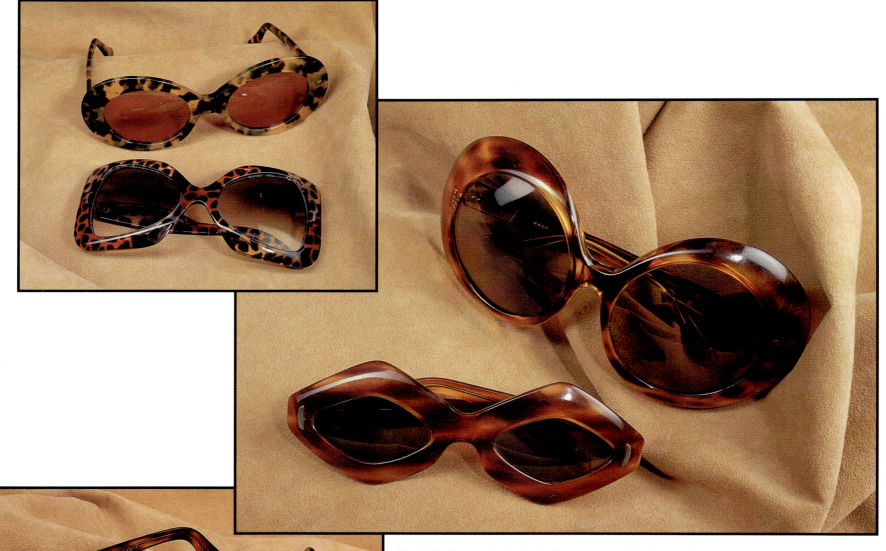

Top left: Two pair of plastic frames, one with leopard spots on translucent orange, yellow and clear background, marked France; the other marked as tortoiseshell, marked Made in USA. Courtesy of Helaine Fendelman.

Above: Two pair of plastic tortoise frames: deep frames marked Made in Italy; diamond-shaped frames unmarked. Courtesy of Helaine Fendelman.

Left: Thick brown tortoiseshell plastic eyewear marked A-S Frame France. Courtesy of Barbara Blau. $35.

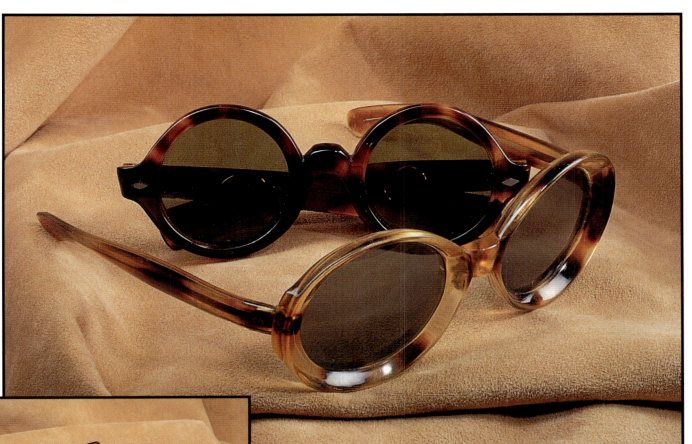

Two pair of plastic tortoiseshell frames: lighter frames marked Made in Italy; darker frames marked Frame France. Courtesy of Helaine Fendelman.

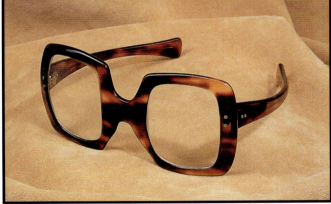

Large and deep tortoiseshell colored plastic frames around square clear lenses, marked Doscar, France. Courtesy of Helaine Fendelman.

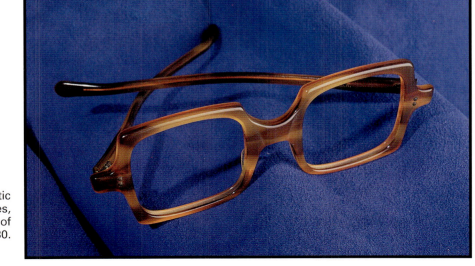

Light tortoiseshell plastic eyewear with square lenses, marked USA. Courtesy of Barbara Blau. $30.

Right: Polygon eyeglasses in two colors of tortoiseshell. Oliver Goldsmith Eyewear Ltd.

Bottom left: Tortoiseshell plastic frames with touches of blue, marked Art Craft USA. Courtesy of Helaine Fendelman.

Bottom right: Blue and white plastic frames with shaded lenses, marked Made in France. Courtesy of Aida's Antiques. $55.

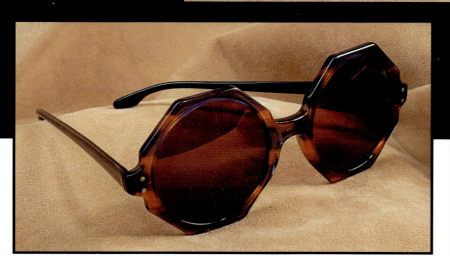

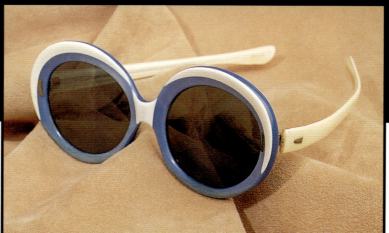

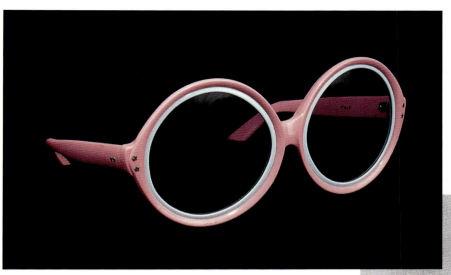

Left: Large pink plastic frames with blue rims around round lenses, marked Italy, and with paper label Samco Italy. Courtesy of Helaine Fendelman.

Below: Black frames with white edge around the circular blue lenses, marked Swank Italy. Courtesy of Helaine Fendelman.

Bottom: Silver plastic eyewear with rounded lenses, marked USA. Courtesy of Barbara Blau. $35.

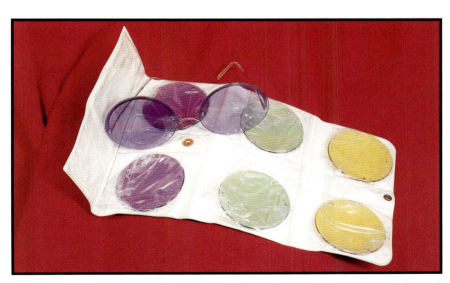

Wire rims with interchangeable large round domed lenses in pale shades of blue, purple, green, and yellow, unmarked. Courtesy of Helaine Fendelman.

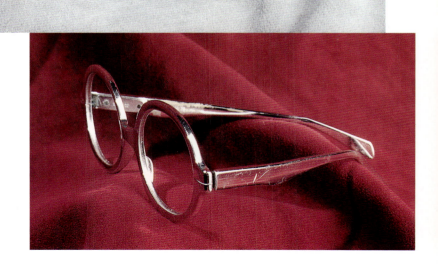

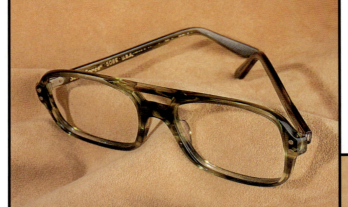

Left: Green translucent plastic frames marked "Solar Spree," USA K+H. Courtesy of Barbara Blau. $25.

Below: Light brown pearl plastic frames around large squared lenses, marked Anglo American Optical Frame England, Mod 101 56x20 LA. Courtesy of Helaine Fendelman.

By the late 1970s, frames became popular with both plain wire rims called "granny glasses" (because they looked like styles your grandparents wore) as well as fancy frames lavishly decorated with rhinestones.

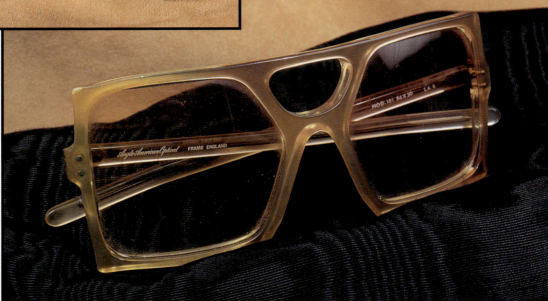

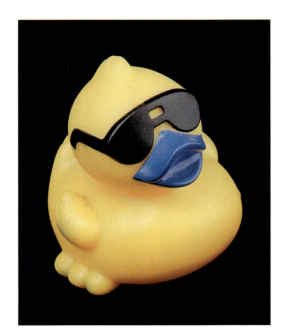

Yellow rubber duck toy with black sunglasses, unmarked. Courtesy of Helaine Fendelman.

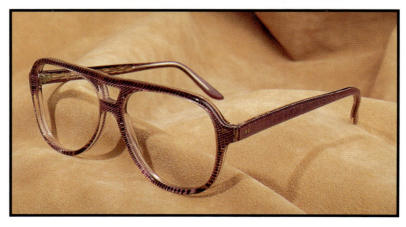

Purple and clear patterned plastic frames with metal supports inside the side pieces, marked V 5 1/2. Courtesy of Barbara Blau.

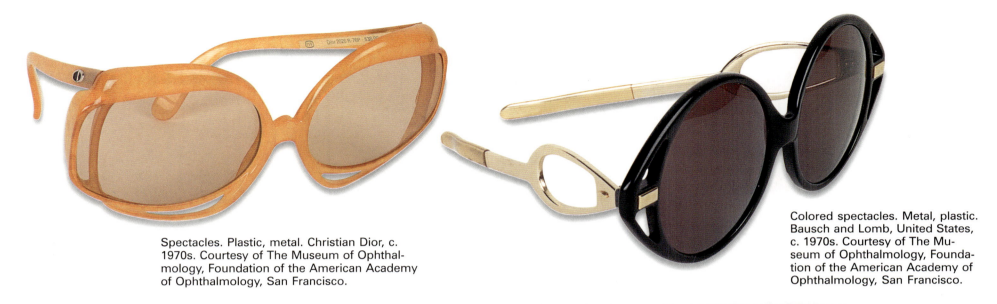

Spectacles. Plastic, metal. Christian Dior, c. 1970s. Courtesy of The Museum of Ophthalmology, Foundation of the American Academy of Ophthalmology, San Francisco.

Colored spectacles. Metal, plastic. Bausch and Lomb, United States, c. 1970s. Courtesy of The Museum of Ophthalmology, Foundation of the American Academy of Ophthalmology, San Francisco.

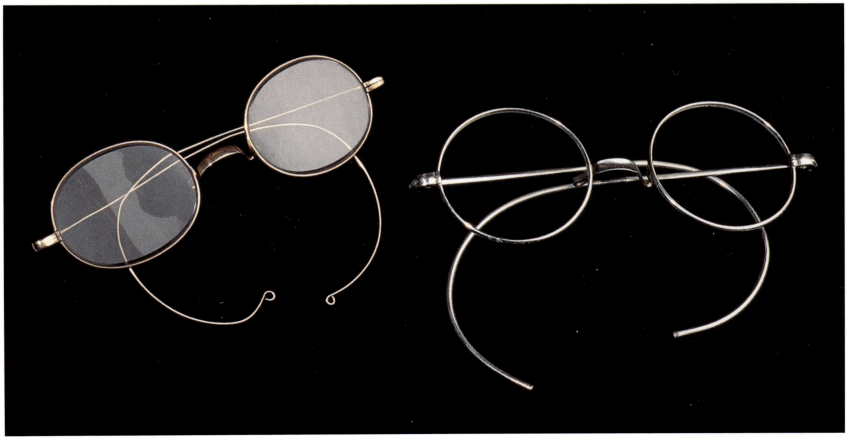

Two pair of eyewear. One silver wire rim frames with curving earpieces. $35. Other small gold wire rims with curved earpieces and looped ends. Courtesy of Barbara Blau. $45.

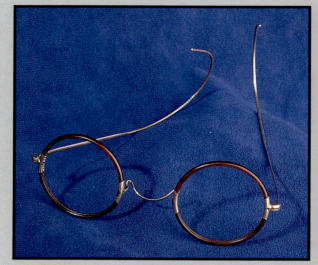
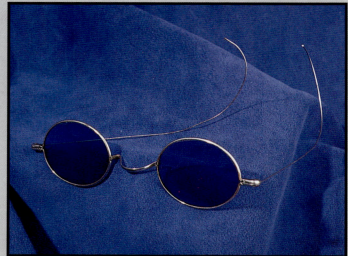
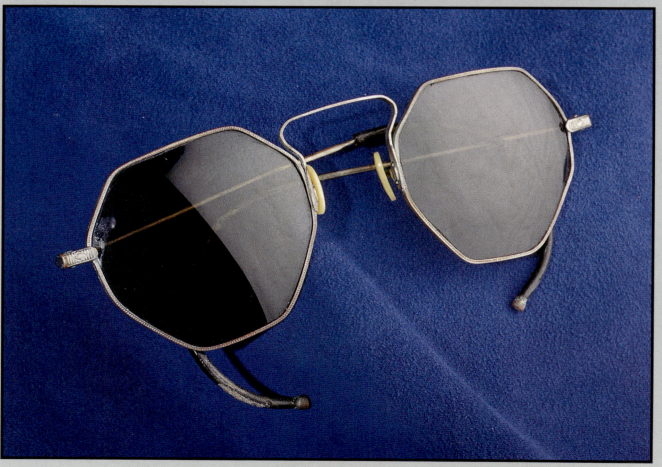

Top left: Brown plastic eyewear with gold metal bridge and side pieces and round lenses. Courtesy of Barbara Blau. $75.

Top right: Silver wire frame eyewear with blue glass lenses and bent wire ear pieces. Courtesy of Barbara Blau. $75.

Right: Gray metal eyewear with gray glass lenses of octagonal shape and curved ear pieces. Courtesy of Barbara Blau. $35.

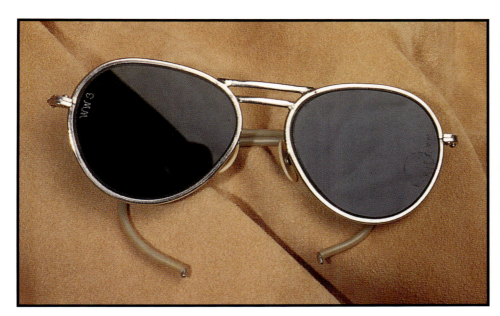

Above: Old green shaded lenses in silver plastic frames and metal side pieces with tubular wrapping, glass marked "WW3" at outside edges. Courtesy of Barbara Blau.

Below: Black plastic eyewear marked Variety-Libra, Frame France. Courtesy of Barbara Blau. $30.

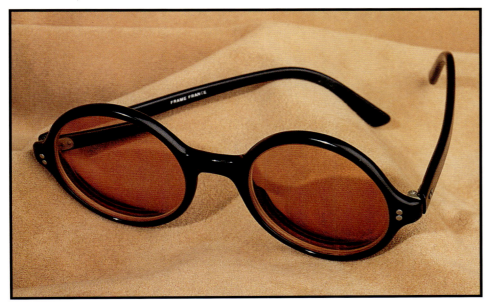

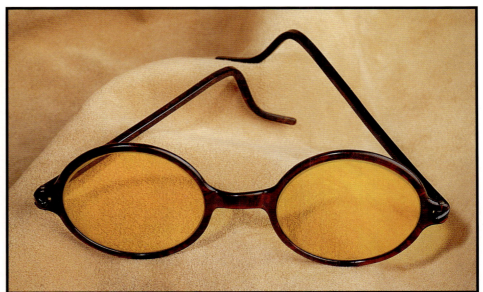

Above: Round brown plastic frames and green glass lenses with unusually shaped ear pieces. Courtesy of Barbara Blau. $45.

Below: Red anodized aluminum frames around round lenses, marked S USA. U.S. Pat. No. 3,243,248. Courtesy of Helaine Fendelman

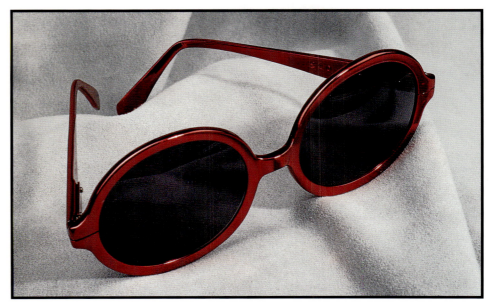

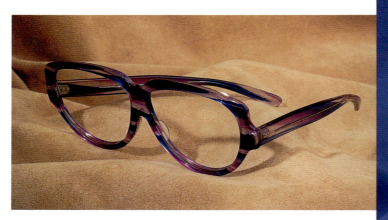

Blue and purple streaked plastic eyewear marked "Lynwood," Bausch & Lomb USA. Courtesy of Barbara Blau. $55.

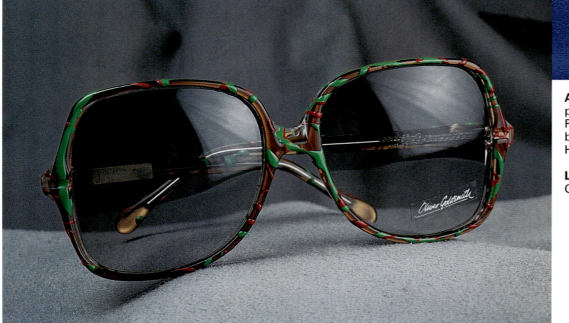

Above: Multicolored and black plastic round frames marked Emilio Pucci, Made in France, with light blue leather slip case. Courtesy of Helaine Fendelman.

Left: Paint drip, acetate. Oliver Goldsmith Eyewear Ltd.

Silver plastic frames around square lenses, black lines in the border, marked Universal 5 1/2. Courtesy of Helaine Fendelman.

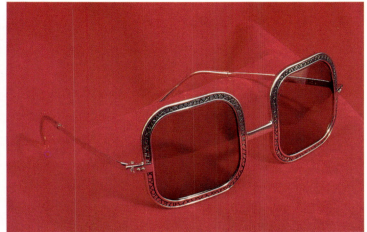

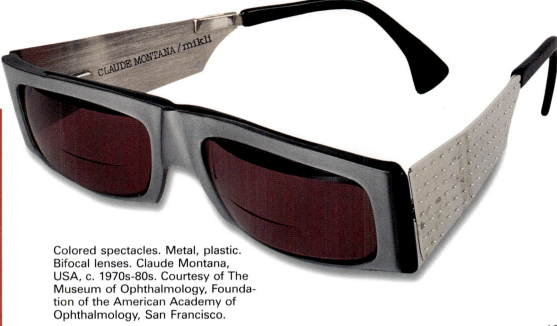

Colored spectacles. Metal, plastic. Bifocal lenses. Claude Montana, USA, c. 1970s-80s. Courtesy of The Museum of Ophthalmology, Foundation of the American Academy of Ophthalmology, San Francisco.

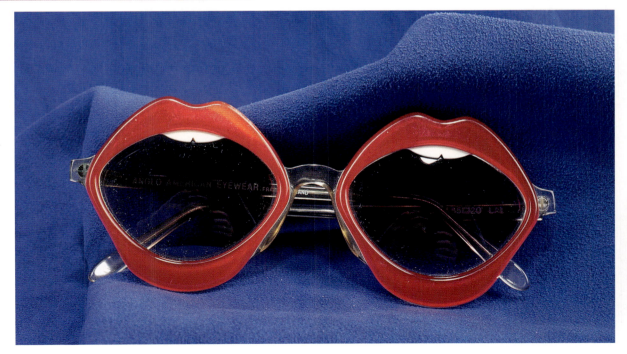

Layered plastic frames in the shape of an open mouth marked Anglo American Eyewear Frame England, Lips 55 (square) 20 LA1. Courtesy of Helaine Fendelman.

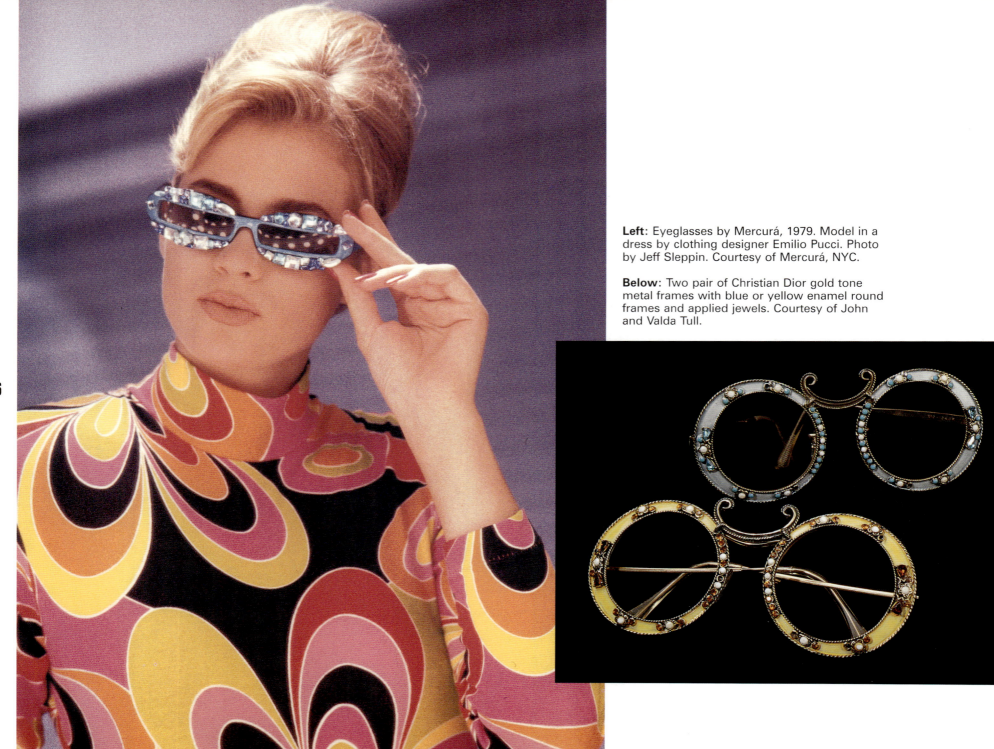

Left: Eyeglasses by Mercurá, 1979. Model in a dress by clothing designer Emilio Pucci. Photo by Jeff Sleppin. Courtesy of Mercurá, NYC.

Below: Two pair of Christian Dior gold tone metal frames with blue or yellow enamel round frames and applied jewels. Courtesy of John and Valda Tull.

Molded polycarbonate plastics were used to make wrap-around frames in 1980, as fashion continued to dominate the shape and function of sunglasses.

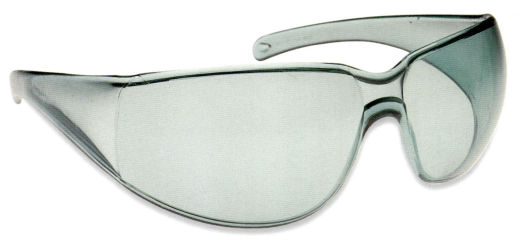

Above: Luna 2, c. 1980, polycarbonate, injection molded green translucent wrap-around style, right arm marked FRANCE. Left arm marked BREVETE PAT. PEND. Oliver Goldsmith Eyewear Ltd.

Right: Nose Guard polycarbonate plastic eyeglasses with wrap-around sides, c. 1980. Oliver Goldsmith Eyewear Ltd.

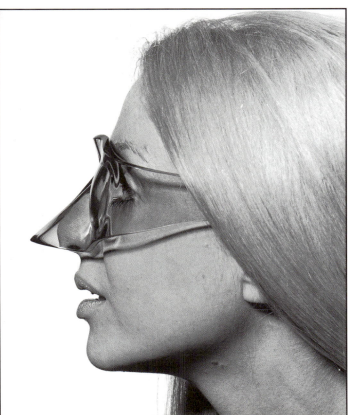

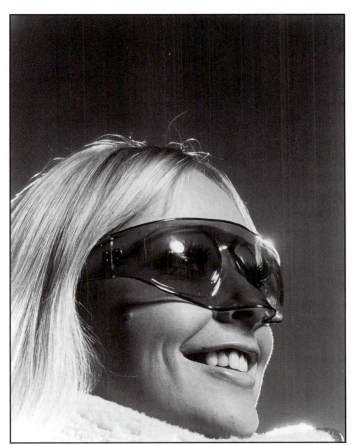

Left: Polycarbonate plastic molded Nose Guard eyeglasses, c. 1980, with hinged sides. Oliver Goldsmith Eyewear Ltd.

Below: Nose Guard polycarbonate plastic eyeglasses, injection molded, c. 1980. Oliver Goldsmith Eyewear Ltd.

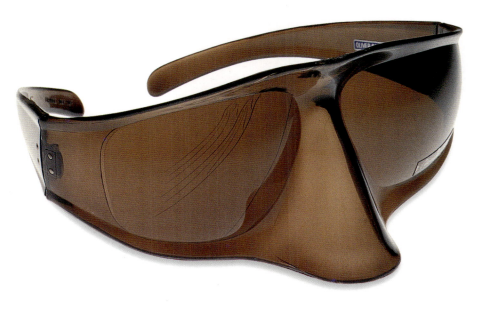

In the 1980s and 1990s, custom order novelty styles were decorated with unconventional trim to create mask-like eyewear meant primarily to cause a sensation. These styles were prominently featured in glamour and publicity photographs and had an effect on the general eyewear market as well. Frames were made to represent animals, birds, and special themes, and they enjoyed a limited popularity on the marketplace. Many companies in Europe and America turned to manufacturers in China, Taiwan, and Japan to produce trendy styles at low cost. Prices became very competitive and advertising budgets soared to capture the "name brand" market worldwide.

New Punk, acetate, c. 1980.
Oliver Goldsmith Eyewear Ltd.

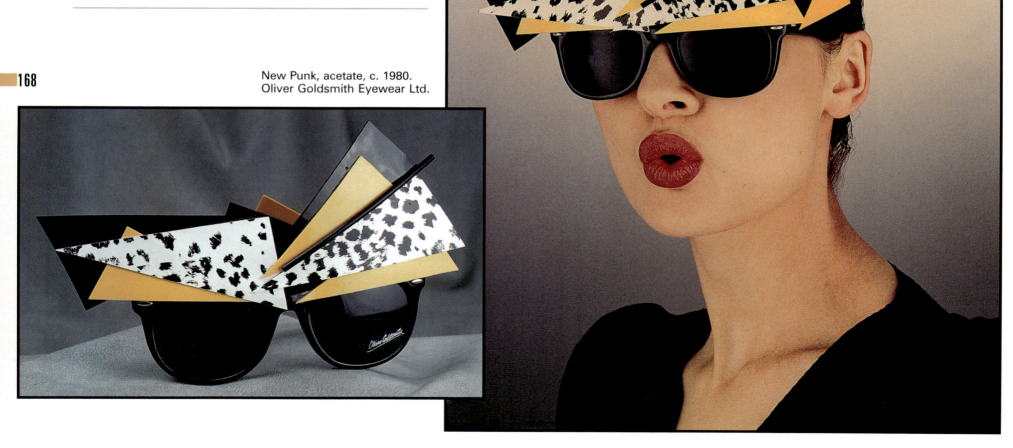

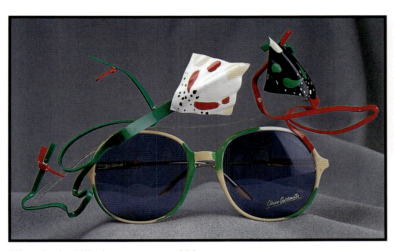

Kites in the Wind, acetate, c. 1980.
Oliver Goldsmith Eyewear Ltd.

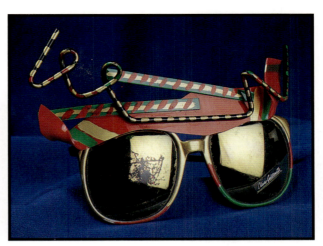

Fantasy 20, acetate eyeglasses, c. 1985. Oliver Goldsmith Eyewear Ltd.

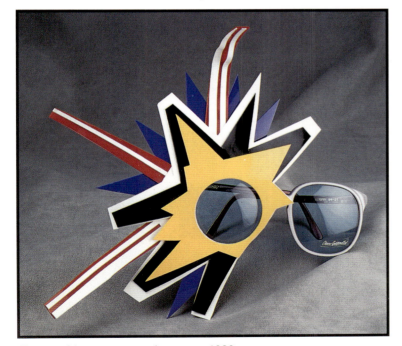

Fantasy 21, acetate eyeglasses, c. 1980.
Oliver Goldsmith Eyewear Ltd.

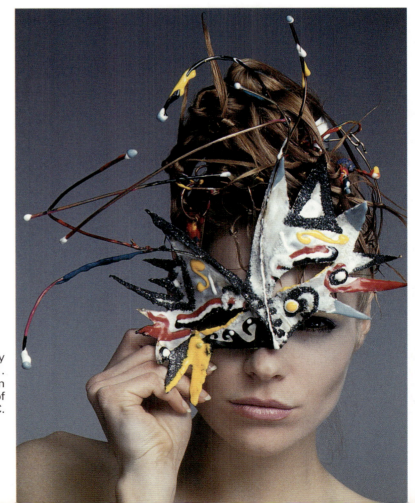

Eyewear by Mercurá, c. 1981. Photo by Norman Isaacs. Courtesy of Mercurá, NYC.

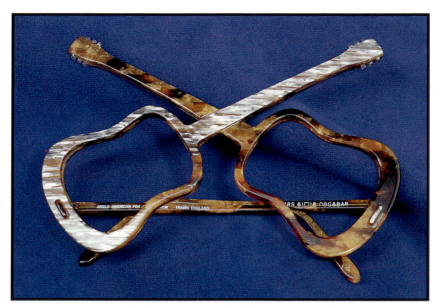

Crossing guitars, Anglo American for Sir Winston Frame England, Guitars 61(square)18 DBG&BAR. Courtesy of Helaine Fendelman.

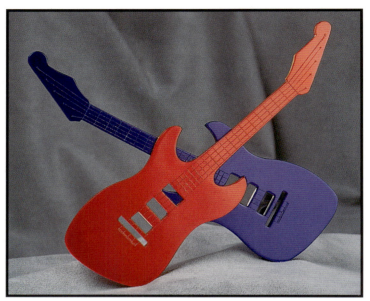

Two Guitars acetate eyeglasses, c. 1985. Oliver Goldsmith Eyewear Ltd.

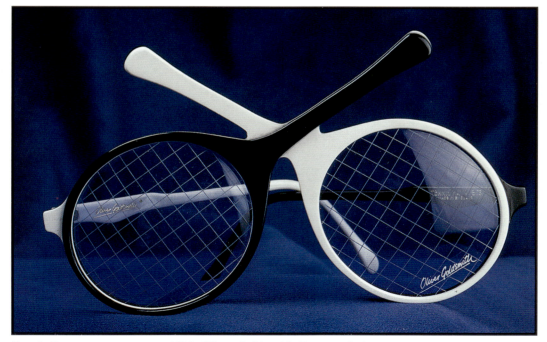

Tennis Racquets, acetate, c. 1982. Oliver Goldsmith Eyewear Ltd.

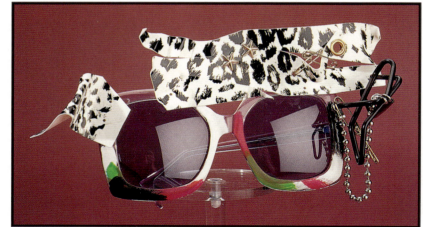

Fantasy 21 "Punk," c.1980-1985, blue translucent frames with painted colors and pins, chain, attachments. Right arm marked Fantasy 7. Left arm marked INCA. Oliver Goldsmith Eyewear Ltd.

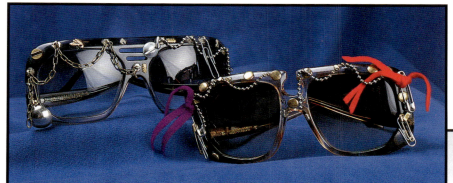

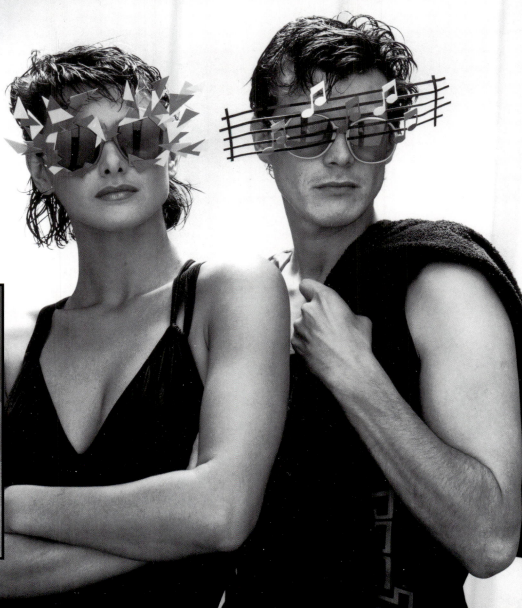

Above: Punk, acetate, c. 1985. Oliver Goldsmith Eyewear Ltd.

Right: Punk eyeglasses and Music Notes eyeglasses, 1985. Oliver Goldsmith Eyewear Ltd.

Below: Music Notes, acetate, c. 1985. Oliver Goldsmith Eyewear Ltd.

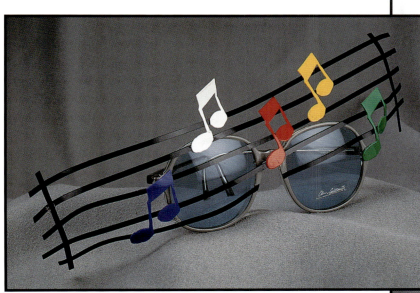

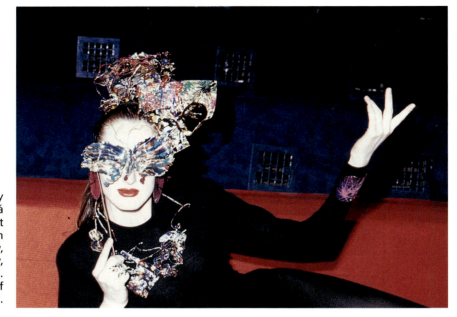

Eyewear by Mercurá displayed at the Palladium fashion show, New York City, in 1988. Courtesy of Mercurá, NYC.

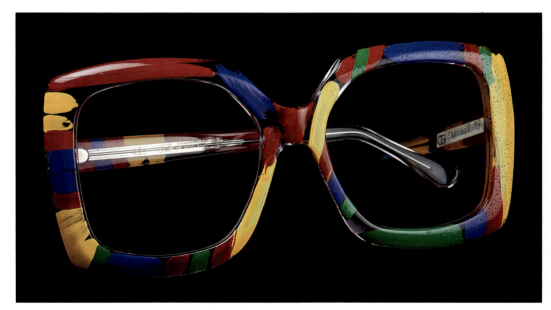

Fantasy 19 eyeglasses, acetate, c. 1985. Oliver Goldsmith Eyewear Ltd.

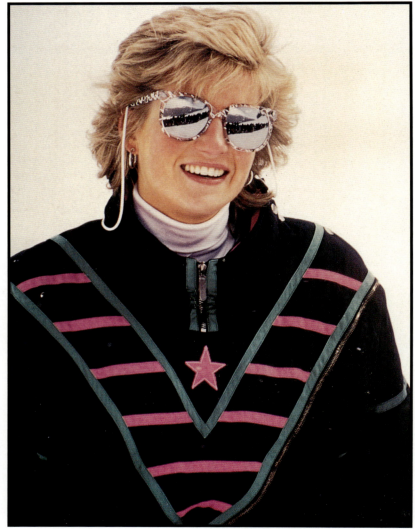

Princess Diana of England wearing acetate eyewear by Oliver Goldsmith, 1985. Oliver Goldsmith Eyewear Ltd.

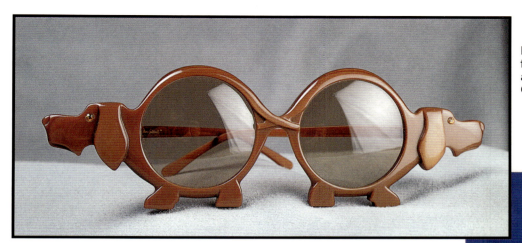

Prototype brown dog frames with tinted lenses, acetate, c. 1985. Oliver Goldsmith Eyewear Ltd.

Black and white dog frames, acetate, c. 1985. Oliver Goldsmith Eyewear Ltd.

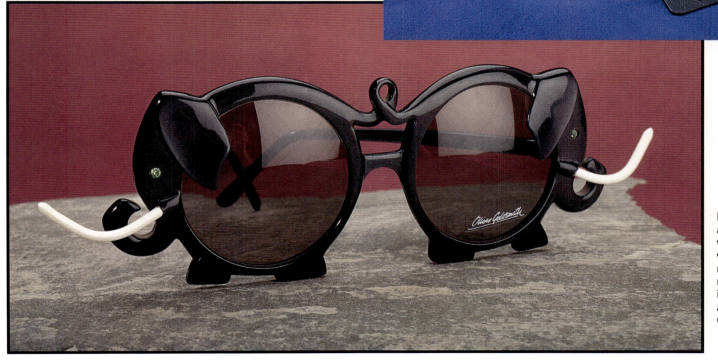

Elephants, c. 1985, acetate black frame with elephant sides and white tusks, green rhinestone eyes. The range in this style also included ducks, storks, and dogs. Oliver Goldsmith Eyewear Ltd.

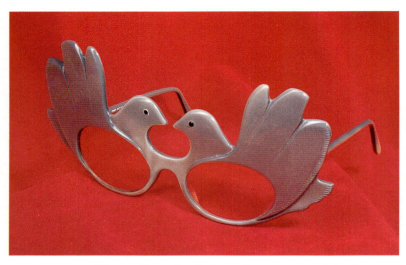

Above: Gray plastic doves frames marked Anglo American Optical Frames France, 1985. *Courtesy of Helaine Fendelman.*

Right: White stork frames with shaded blue lenses, designed for England's Princess Diana, c. 1985. Oliver Goldsmith Eyewear Ltd.

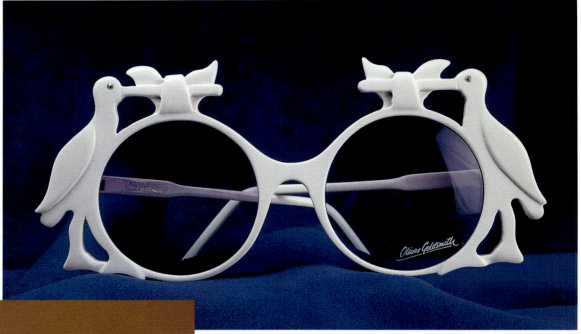

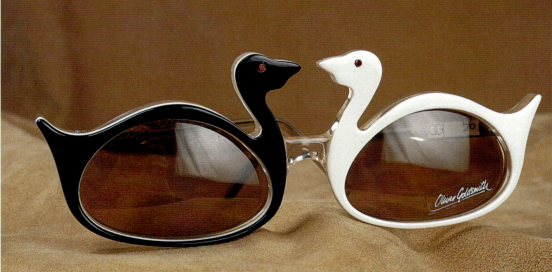

Above: Ducks eyeglasses, acetate, c. 1985. Oliver Goldsmith Eyewear Ltd.

Right: White ducks frames, c. 1985, marked Anglo American Frame England, Mod Swan 55 (square) 20. Courtesy of Helaine Fendelman.

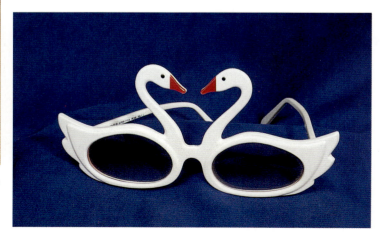

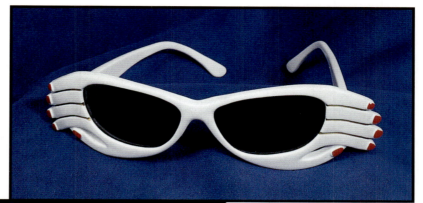

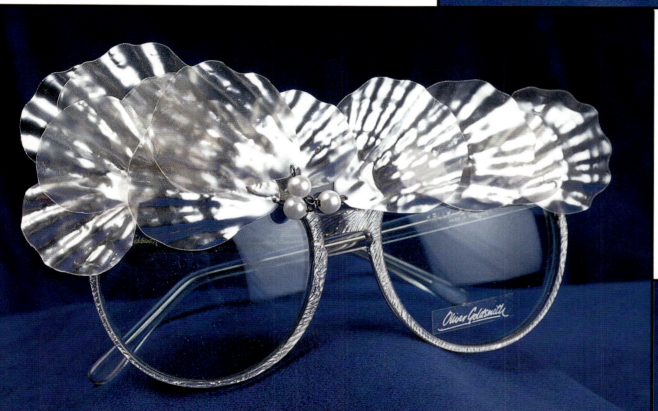

Above: White frame with hands and red painted nails, c. 1985, marked Korea. Courtesy of Helaine Fendelman.

Left: Pearl shells above tinted lenses, acetate, c. 1985. Oliver Goldsmith Eyewear Ltd.

Below: Pink frames with holly leaf and berry ornaments and maroon temples, acetate, c. 1985. Oliver Goldsmith Eyewear Ltd.

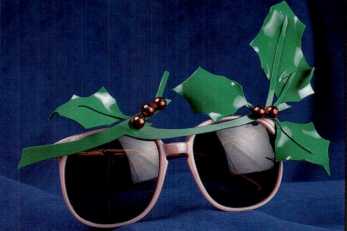

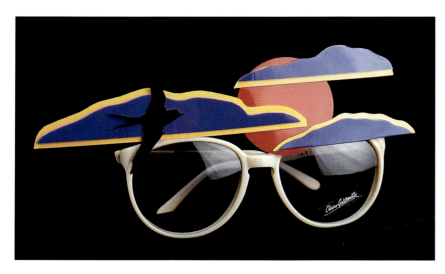

Above: Fantasy eyeglasses with tinted lenses, acetate, c. 1985. Oliver Goldsmith Eyewear Ltd.

Right: Sunglasses and hair accessories by Mercurá, 1989. Photo by Frank Franca. Courtesy of Mercurá, NYC.

Below: Black frames decorated with rhinestones, signed Jan Carlen, '89, Taiwan R.O.C. Courtesy of Helaine Fendelman.

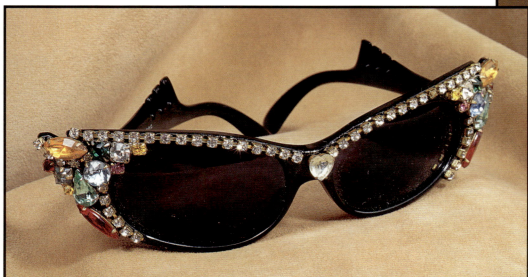

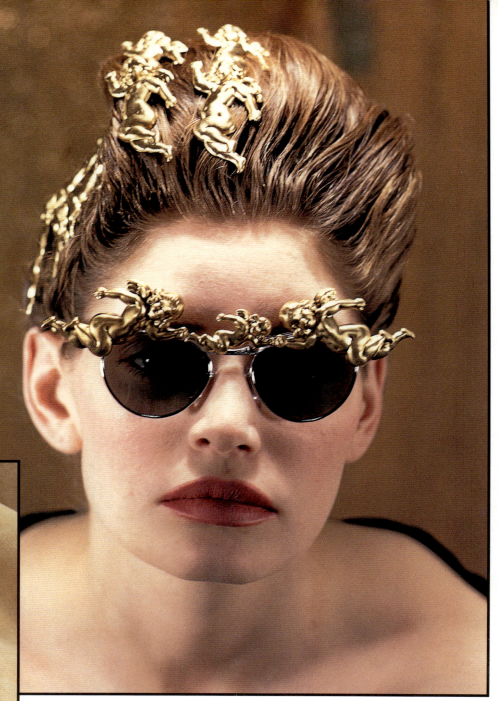

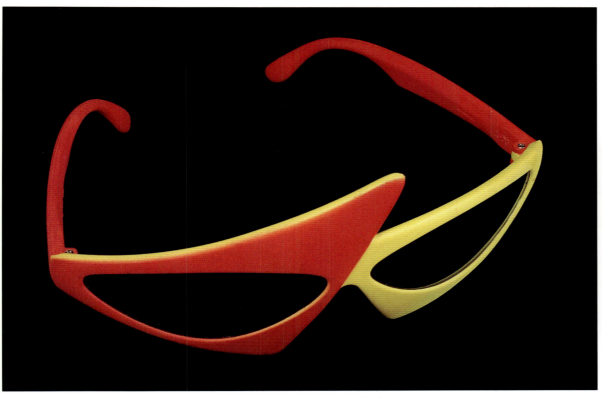

Asymmetrical frames of orange and yellow soft plastic marked © 1989 PHI, Taiwan 1-05. Courtesy of Helaine Fendelman.

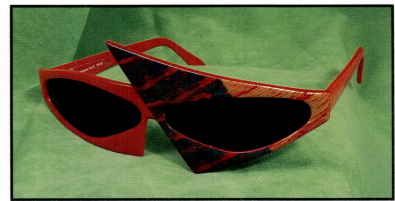

Modern red plastic with asymmetrical frames, one jagged side painted with brushed lines, marked Taiwan ROC. Courtesy of Helaine Fendelman.

177

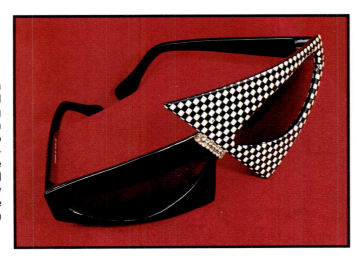

Black plastic with asymmetrical frames, a jutting side painted with white squares, two rows of rhinestones on the nose pieces, marked Taiwan. Courtesy of Helaine Fendelman

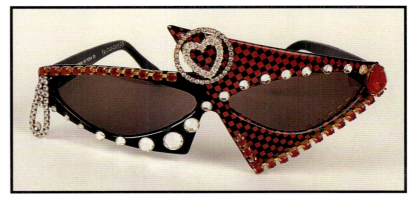

Colored Spectacles. Plastic, rhinestones. Jan Carlen, Taiwan, c. 1989-90. Courtesy of The Museum of Ophthalmology, Foundation of the American Academy of Ophthalmology, San Francisco.

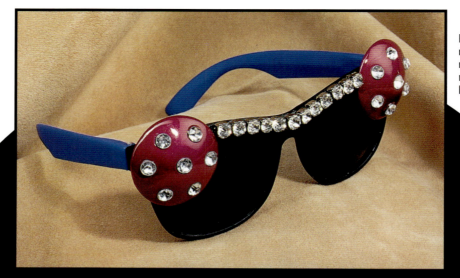

Black frames decorated with two red discs (buttons?) and clear rhinestones, blue soft plastic arms marked Taiwan. Courtesy of Helaine Fendelman.

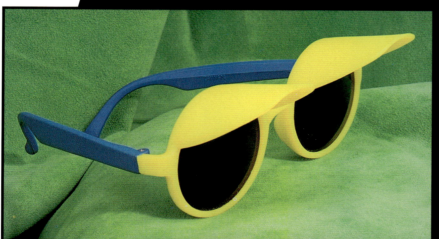

Soft plastic molded with yellow visor over the lenses, blue arms molded Taiwan, 3-14, ©1989 PHI. Courtesy of Helaine Fendelman.

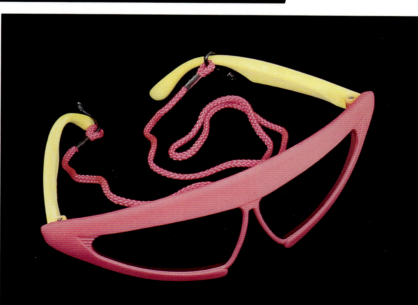

Dark pink soft plastic frames with yellow arms marked ©1989 PHI. Courtesy of Helaine Fendelman

Right: Sunglasses by Mercurá, 1990. Photo by Michel Turolla. Courtesy of Mercurá, NYC.

Below: Sunglasses by Mercurá, 1990. Photo by Tim Goetz. Courtesy of Mercurá, NYC.

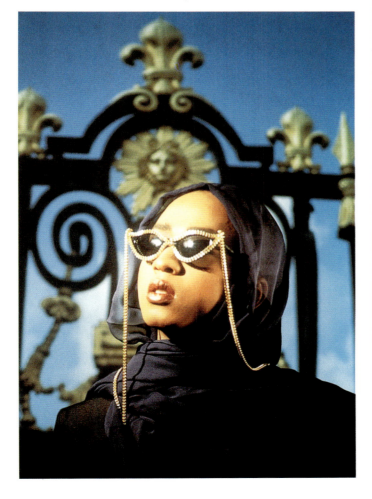

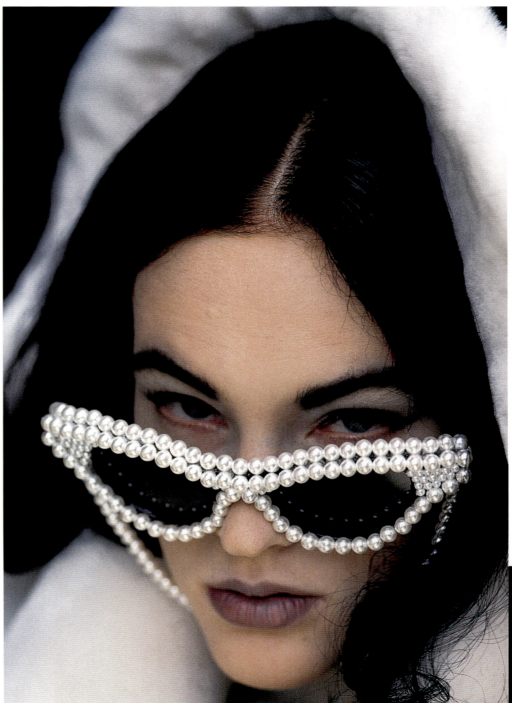

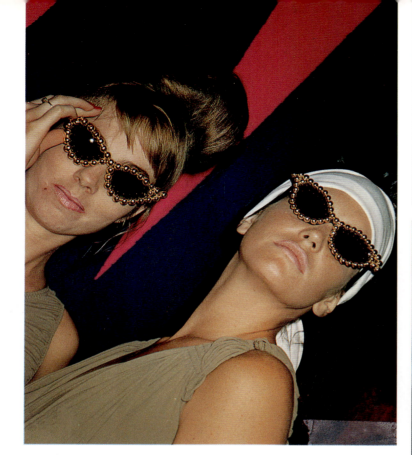

Left: Sunglasses by Mercurá, 1990. Courtesy of Mercurá, NYC.

Lower left: Sunglasses by Mercurá, 1991. Courtesy of Mercurá, NYC.

Below: Sunglasses by Mercurá, 1991. Courtesy of Mercurá, NYC.

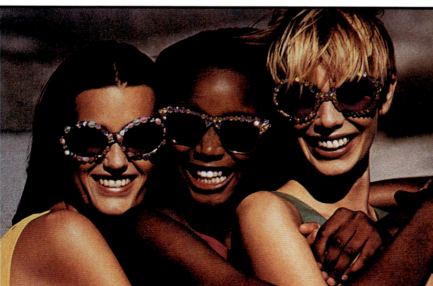

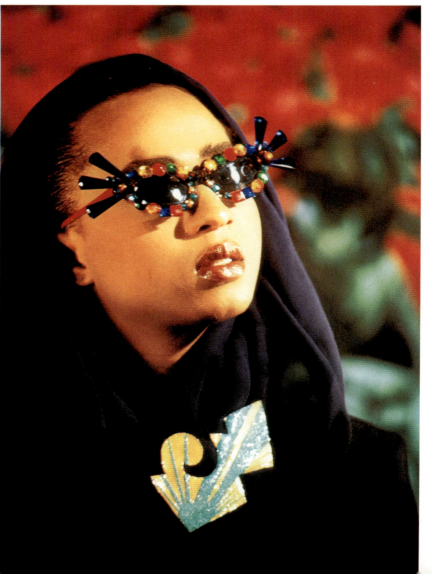

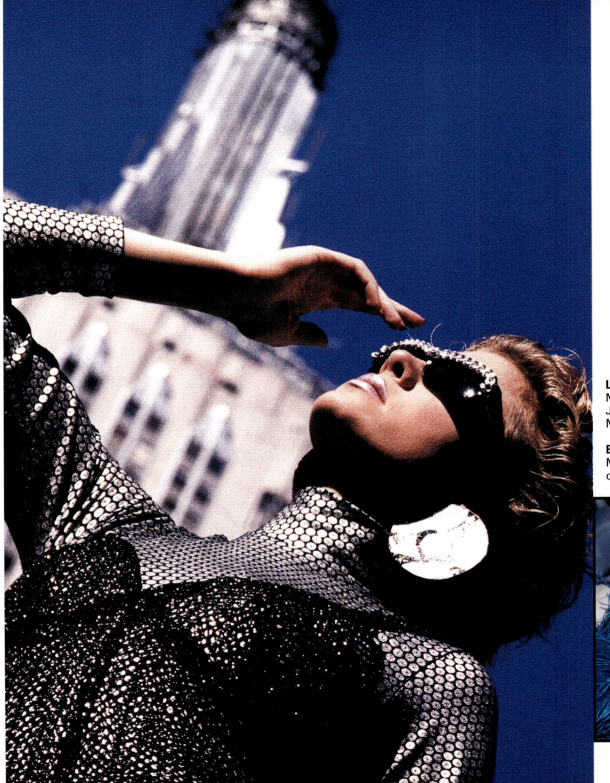

Left: Sunglasses by Mercurá, 1991. Photo by Jeff Sleppin. Courtesy of Mercurá, NYC.

Below: Sunglasses by Mercurá, 1992. Courtesy of Mercurá, NYC.

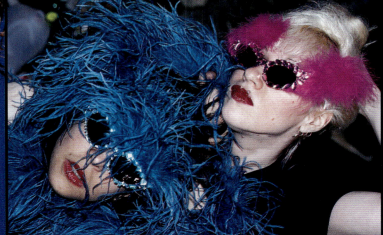

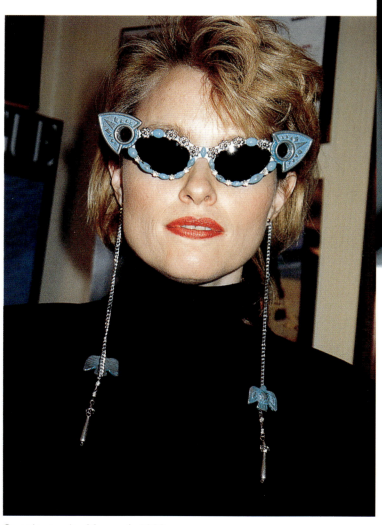

Sunglasses by Mercurá, 1992.
Courtesy of Mercurá, NYC.

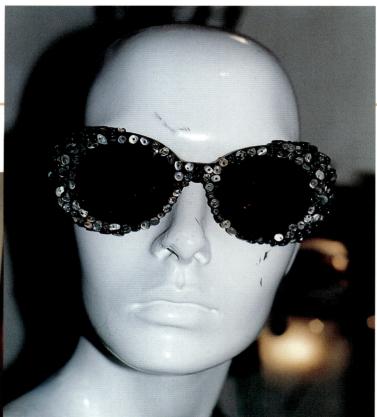

Left: Sunglasses by Mercurá, 1992. Courtesy of Mercurá, NYC.

Below: Sunglasses by Mercurá, 1993. Courtesy of Mercurá, NYC.

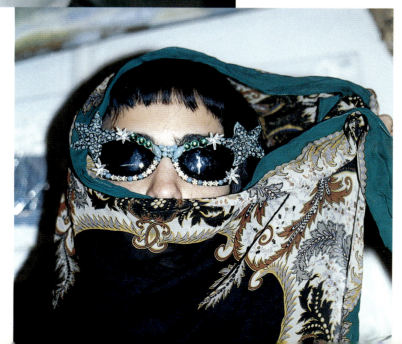

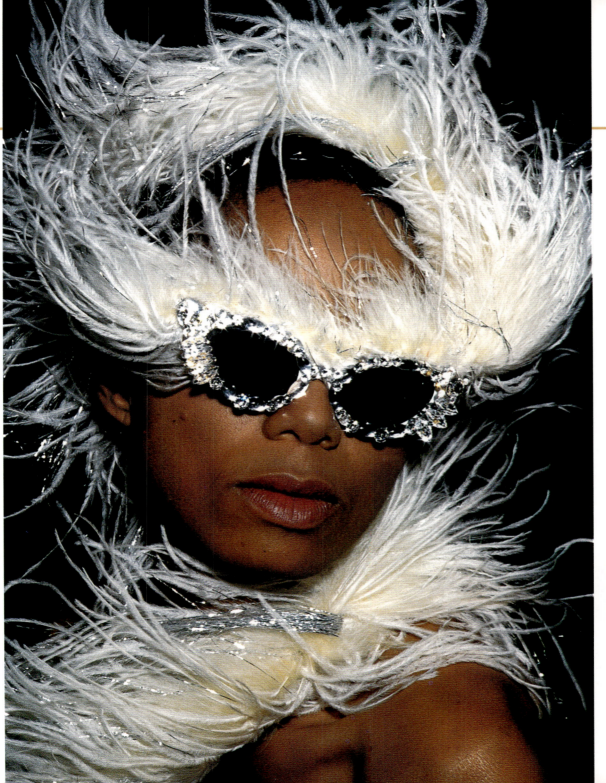

Sunglasses by Mercurá, 1995. Photo by Paula Retsky. Courtesy of Mercurá, NYC.

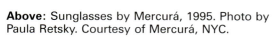

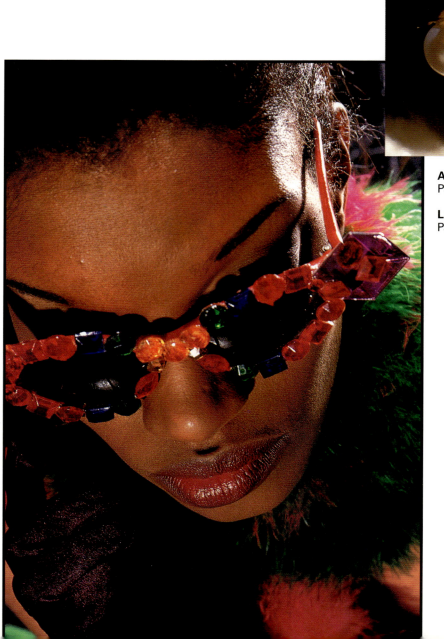

Above: Sunglasses by Mercurá, 1995. Photo by Paula Retsky. Courtesy of Mercurá, NYC.

Left: Sunglasses by Mercurá, 1995. Photo by Paula Retsky. Courtesy of Mercurá, NYC.

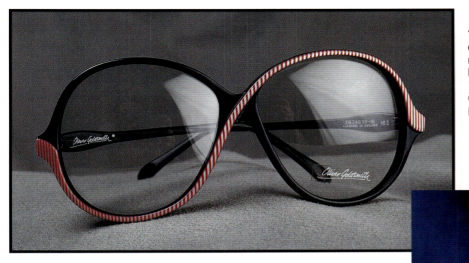

"Zig-zag" eyeglasses with red stripe on blue, acetate, 1985. Oliver Goldsmith Eyewear Ltd.

All the while, conservative styles also were selling widely in the commercial fashion market. New materials, such as lightweight but very strong titanium, were used for frames to achieve very sleek styles. By the end of the 1990s, eyewear designs made simply for fun, some even without any lenses at all, were created and sold in the variety market.

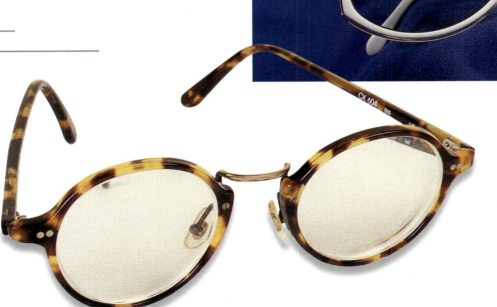

Above: "Berwick," c. 1986, (as worn by Princess Diana) acetate white thin frame. Oliver Goldsmith Eyewear Ltd.

Left: Spectacles. Plastic. Calvin Klein, Italy, 1980–90. Courtesy of The Museum of Ophthalmology, Foundation of the American Academy of Ophthalmology, San Francisco.

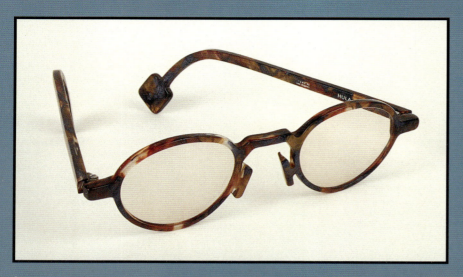
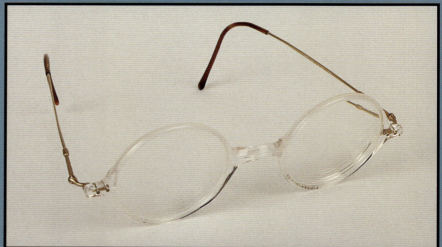
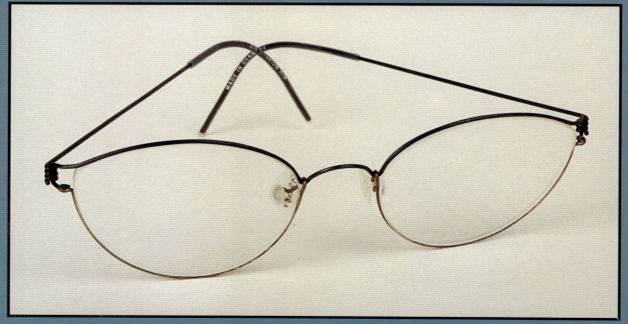

Above left: Spectacles. Plastic. L.A. Eyeworks, USA/Italy, c. 1980s-90s. Courtesy of The Museum of Ophthalmology, Foundation of the American Academy of Ophthalmology, San Francisco.

Above right: Spectacles. Plastic, metal. Giorgio Armani, Italy, c. 1990s. Courtesy of The Museum of Ophthalmology, Foundation of the American Academy of Ophthalmology, San Francisco.

Right: Spectacles. Metal, plastic. Frame made of wire using no screws. "Air Titanium rim". Denmark, c. 1980s-90s. Courtesy of The Museum of Ophthalmology, Foundation of the American Academy of Ophthalmology, San Francisco.

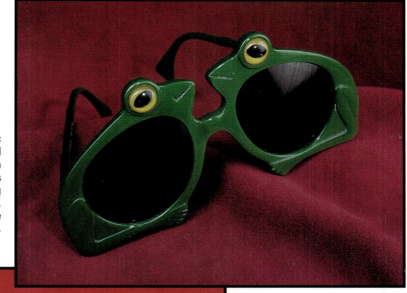

Green frog plastic frames marked Anglo American Eyewear Frames England, Frog 50(square)20 SO3. Courtesy of Helaine Fendelman.

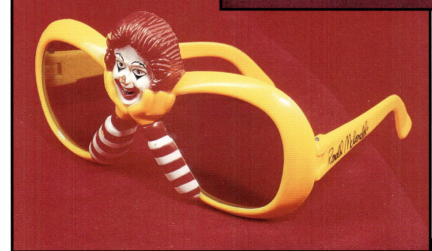

Yellow plastic with Ronald McDonald face and hands on the bridge, one arm signed Ronald McDonald, other arm marked © McDonald's Made in China PW. Courtesy of Helaine Fendelman

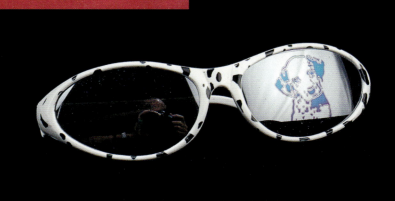

White plastic frames with black spots around silvered lenses printed with a Dalmatian's head, marked © Disney's 101 Dalmatians, pan oceanic ® Taiwan. Courtesy of Helaine Fendelman.

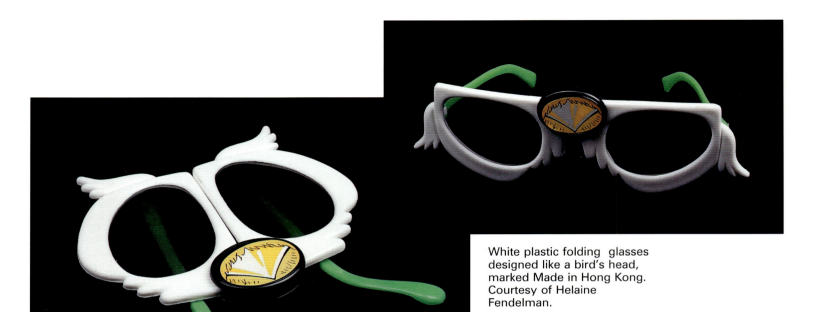

White plastic folding glasses designed like a bird's head, marked Made in Hong Kong. Courtesy of Helaine Fendelman.

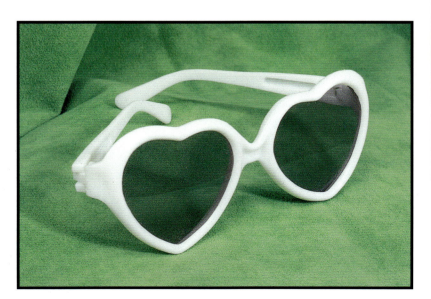

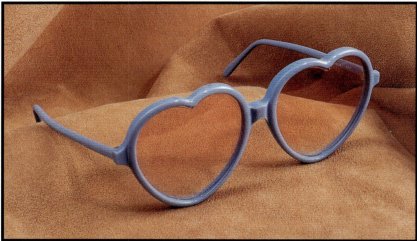

Above: Light blue heart-shaped frames marked Anglo American Optical Frame England, Mod Heart 55x16 SO9. Courtesy of Helaine Fendelman

Left: Modern white soft plastic frames with heart shape around the lenses, unmarked. Courtesy of Helaine Fendelman.

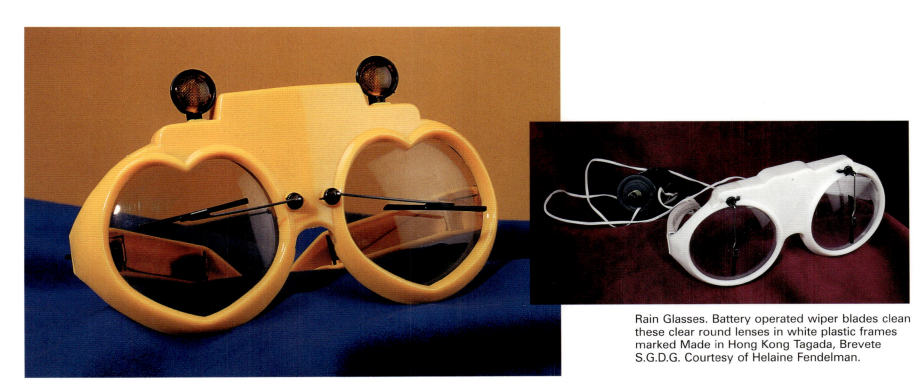

Yellow plastic frames with battery powered mechanism to operate wipers and lights over the heart-shaped frames, unmarked. Courtesy of John and Valda Tull.

Rain Glasses. Battery operated wiper blades clean these clear round lenses in white plastic frames marked Made in Hong Kong Tagada, Brevete S.G.D.G. Courtesy of Helaine Fendelman.

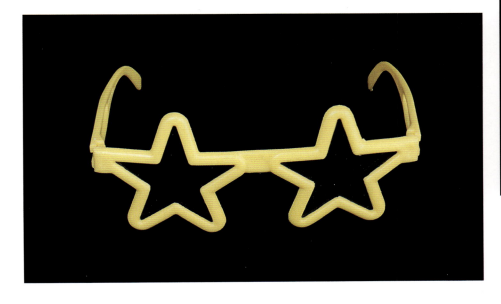

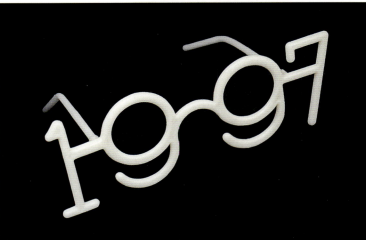

Above: Happy New Year! Molded white plastic frames designed as 1997, no lenses, unmarked. Courtesy of Helaine Fendelman

Left: Yellow plastic frames around star-shaped lenses, marked Made in China. Courtesy of Helaine Fendelman.

CONCLUSION

From science to fashion, the eyewear field has evolved with designs of interest for everyone. Where will the new millennium take the industry? Definitely to the limits of knowledge and imagination. Far out there.

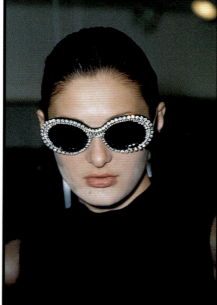

Sunglasses for Vera Wang Couture by Mercurá, 1997. Photo by Greg Kitchen. Courtesy of Mercurá, NYC.

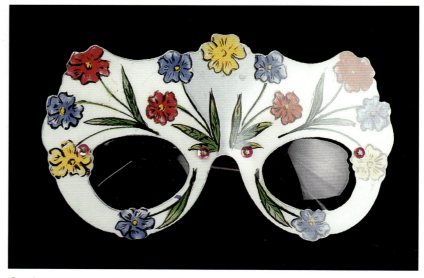

Garden party eyeglasses, acetate. Oliver Goldsmith Eyewear Ltd.

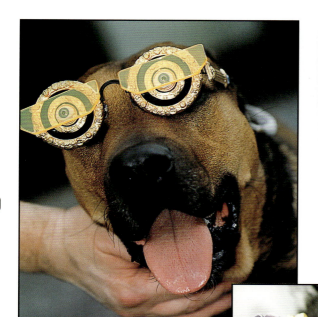

Above & right: Eyewear by Mercurá, 1998. Courtesy of Mercurá, NYC.

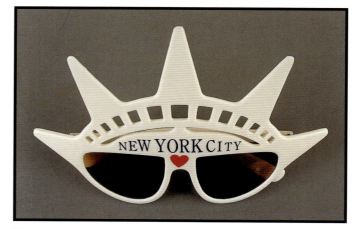

White plastic Statue of Liberty design sunglasses, souvenir of New York, 1999. Private collection

BIBLIOGRAPHY

Andressen, B. Michael. *Spectacles, From Utility Article to Cult Object*. Stuttgart: Arnoldsche, 1998.

Corson, Richard. *Fashions in Eyeglasses, from the 14th century to the present day*. London: Peter Owen Limited, 1967.

Leach, Alan. *Old English Patents for Spectacles from 1783 until the end of the 19th century*. Halifax, West Yorkshire, U. K.: Ophthalmic Antiques International Collectors' Club, 1998.

Macgregor, Ronald J. S., ed. *Ophthalmic Antiques Extracts 1986-1996*. West Kilbride, Ayrshire, U.K.: The Ophthalmic Antiques International Collectors' Club, 1996.

Monique. "Paris plays frameup game," *New York Sunday News*. New York, July 25, 1971.

On the Nose: Eyeglasses in New York. Exhibition. New York: The New York Historical Society, October 15, 1997 to January 11, 1998.

Perec, Georges, and Yves Hersant, photgraphy by Timothy Street-Porter. "Hollywood on Eyes," *FMR America*. August 1984, #3, p. 95.

Rosenthal, J. William, M.D. *Spectacles and Other Vision Aids, A History and Guide to Collecting*. San Francisco: Norman Publishing, 1996.

INDEX

101Dalmatians spectacles, 187
1997 spectacles, 189
A-S, 156
Abraham, Albert, 60
Adams, George, 26, 51
Adelaide spectacle, 85
advertising card, 41, 46, 50, 58, 59, 62, 70, 78, 91, 107, 114, 124
ai tai lens, 12, 15
Air Titanium rim, 186
Allan Optical, 153
aluminum case, 75
aluminum frames, 111, 115, 116, 130
amber lens, 30
amblyopia glasses, 77
America Optical Company, 93, 95, 98, 108, 110
Anglo American Eyewear, 165, 170, 187
Anglo American Optical, 121, 129, 160, 174, 188
Appo spectacles, 123
Armani, Giorgio, 186
Art Craft, 158
Artist spectacle, 88
Askey, Arthur, 113, 121
Astig clip, 63
asymmetrical frames, 177
Athway, 98
aviator's glasses, 93
Ayscough, James, 18
azurine lens, 89
B & L, 144
Bakelite, 66
baleen frames, 7, 11, 64
Baltimore, 50
Bang-On spectacles, 127
Barnitz, E. A. & Son Jewelers, 79
Bate, Robert Bretell, 51
Bausch & Lomb, 102, 114, 117, 161, 164
Beecher, William, 31
BelAir, 141
Berwick spectacles, 185
bi-concave lens, 20, 33
bifocal lens, 22, 33, 42, 60
billiards glasses, 68
Birmingham, England, 66, 74
Black For-her spectacles, 123
bone frame, 7, 64
Boston pince-nez, 60
Braham, John, 60, 68
brass frame, 12, 13, 18, 26, 27, 32, 59
Brevette, 167
bridge (nosepiece), 2, 12
brille lens, 8

bronze frames, 12
Bull Dog spectacle, 85
Bussey, George, 51
Butterfly spectacles, 120
c-shaped bridge, 18
C.O.C., 112
cable temple, 39
Caine, Michael, 135
Caloban, 96, 98
Capri spectacles, 152
Carlen, Jan, 176, 177
Carnarvonshire, 70
cases, 19
Cassini, Oleg, 132
cataracts, 78
chain temples, 122
chains for eyeglasses, 70
Chance-Pilkington, 124
Chank, J. S., 28
chatelaine, 74
Chelsea Art spectacle, 84, 87
Chinese styles, 7, 12-16
Clent Goldside spectacles, 154
coin silver frame, 42
colored lens, 15, 17-20, 22, 23, 25, 30, 31, 42, 60-63, 65, 67, 68, 70, 72, 78, 89
Comet, 139
Cool Ray, 97, 102
copper case, 32
Corson, Richard, 7
counter display, 78, 81
Courreges, Andre, 126, 132
Cover's Rubber Goggles, 76
Curry, William, 60, 66
Cutts, L. P., 67
Daffy spectacles, 121
Dawn spectacle, 84, 87
Dior, Christian, 132, 154, 161, 166
Disneyland glasses, 107
Dixie spectacles, 152
Dog spectacles, 173
Dors, Diana, 106
Doscar, 157
Doves spectacles, 174
Drew spectacles, 114
driving glasses, 76, 89
Ducks spectacles, 174
Dutch tiles, 9
ear hook, 70
ear trumpet, 51, 57
earpiece, 2
Ekland, Britt, 133
Elephants spectcles, 173
Elfin spectacle, 86

Elkington, George Richards, 22
Emeraldite, 97
Erhard, Johan, 9
Erinoid plastics, 84, 87
Escort Aluminum, 111
Eskimo shade, 64
Eskimo, 7
European styles, 8
Evard, L., 150, 153
fabric case, 16
Fantasy spectacles, 176
Fantasy 7 spectacles, 170
Fantasy 19 spectacles, 172
Fantasy 20 spectacles, 169
Fantasy 21 "Punk" spectacles, 170
Fantasy 21 spectacles, 169
Fehl, Jean, 51
field glass, 36
Flair Originals, 140
FlairNike spectacles, 140
flesh-colored frame, 84
folding temple, 27
Foremost, 139
Franklin, Benjamin, 22
Frawley, John Joseph, 60
Freund Brothers, 62, 96
gas mask glasses, 76
Gaspari, 108
Glasgow, Scotland, 83
Globe Special lens, 63
Goerz, Paul, 60
gold frame, 18, 32, 33, 36, 39, 42, 44, 52-55, 72, 80, 110, 111
Goldsmith, Oliver, 84-88, 95, 106, 132
Goo-Goo-Decor spectacles, 121
granny glasses, 160
gunning glasses, 68
Gutenberg, Johannes, 8
gutta percha eyewear, 72
half-frame glasses, 119
Hall, George, 74
Hanau, 51
Harlequin, 103
Haverhill, Massachusetts, 92
Heath, Charles, 71
Helmecke, 140
hinge, 2, 17, 18
HOE, 141
Holmes, John, 25
Hope spectacles, 123
horn frames, 12, 14, 16, 18, 20, 28, 37, 80
Horon, Marjorie, 114
Huber, Harry D., 47
Hughes, E., 31

Ihne, William Berthold, 68
International Jewelry Co., 92
iron frames, 18
ivory netsuke, 6
J. F. S. Sons, 70
Janvey, H., 25
Jason spectacles, 103
Jester spectacles, 112
k-bridge, 18, 39
K. K. Spectacle Co., 97
Ketcham & McDougall, 70, 71
Kites in the Wind spectacles, 169
Klein, Calvin, 185
Kono Sales Co., 119, 138
L.A. Eyeworks, 186
lacquer frames, 12
lacquered case, 12, 14, 25
LaLunette spectacles, 137
LaScala spectacles, 129
leather case, 19, 25, 29, 36, 38, 44, 45, 48-50, 54, 72
leather frame, 10, 94
Lenheis, 27
lens, 2
Liberty, 120
Library spectacle, 87
Liverpool, 68
lizard skin, 11, 13
Lizars, J. Optician, 83
lorgnette, 17, 26, 51-59, 79, 80, 90, 94, 105, 106
Lubin, Siegmund, 60
Luna 2 spectacles, 167
Luna Overlapped, 103
Lynwood, 164
magnifier, 21, 34
magnifying glasses, 8
mailing box, 50, 91, 92
Manchester, England, 68
marcasite, 90, 111
Mars, 152
Martin's Margins, 20
Martin, Benjamin, 20
master's glasses, 77
May, 153
McAllister & Brother, 40, 45
McAllister & Co., 40
McAllister & Son, 40
McAllister cases, 40-50
McAllister, Francis W., 40, 50
McAllister , J. Cook, 40
McAllister, John, Jr., 40
McAllister, John, Sr., 40, 41
McAllister, John W., 40
McAllister Opt. Co., 40, 46, 47
McAllister Opticians, 33, 40-50
McAllister, Thomas H., 40, 49
McAllister, William Mitchell, 40
McAllister, William Y., 40, 46

McDonald, Ronald spectacles, 187
Mercurá, 166, 169, 172, 176, 179-184, 190
metal case, 13, 82, 83
Metalite, 108
mica lens, 12
Mike spectacles, 136
Milano, 152
Mod Heart spectacles, 188
Mona Lisa spectacles, 110
monocle, 36, 79
monocular, 36
Montana, Claude, 165
Morecambe, Eric, 136
mother-of-pearl case, 35
Moto-glas lens, 89
Mullineux, Matthew, 68
Music notes spectacles, 171
nearsighted lens, 43
Negretti & Zambra, 36
New Punk spectacles, 168
New York, 50, 71, 78
Nose Guard spectacles, 167
numbers inscribed, 34
Nuremberg magnifiers, 8
nylon frame, 105
Ogle spectacles, 146
Oliver Goldsmith Eyewear Ltd., 74, 75, 79, 80, 84-88, 95, 106, 112-114, 120, 121, 123, 124, 127, 128, 132, 133-136, 146, 149, 154, 158, 167-176, 190
OO-er T.V. Specs spectacles, 128
opera glass, 36, 46, 56
Orthogon Lenses, 80
Owen, Jas. W. & Co. Opticians, 72
Oxford pince-nez, 72
Padishell spectacle, 86
paper case, 8, 18, 19, 28, 30, 42
papier maché case, 8, 18
Paxton, George, 66
Peale, Charles Willson, 23
pearl diver glasses, 65
Peck & Peck stores, 133
Peel, D. W., Optometrist, 92
Perfection Spectacles, 78
Perris, Anne Marie, 142
Peters, J., 30
Philadelphia, Penna., 40, 50, 60, 72
Pickard, Joseph Fidoe, 60
pince-nez, 9, 51, 60-63, 66, 72, 73, 79
pivoting temple, 27
plastic frame, 36, 75, 89, 94, 95-190
Plenty, S., 38
Pocket spectacle, 84
Poland spectacle, 86
Polaroid lens, 97, 102
polycarbonate plastics, 167
Polygon spectacle, 158
Portsmouth spectacles, 85
postcard, 58

pounce, 34
Prince spectacles, 84, 87
Princess Grace of Monaco, 123
prism glasses, 33
projector slide, 49, 50
Protecto Shield eyeglasses, 81
Pucci, Emilio, 164, 166
Punk spectacles, 171
Purdom, Robert, 66
Pyramid spectacles, 128
quartz lens, 12, 14
Queen, James W. & Co., 56
Radiant by Universal. 114
railroad glasses, 30, 65-67
Ray-Ban, 102, 114, 144
Raybert, 104
Reading, Pennsylvania, 77
reed frames, 12
respirator goggles, 75
Rich, S., 21
Richardson, John, 22
Rip spectacles, 124
Roberts, David, 70
Roberts, Emilie, 145
Romeo spectacles, 116
Rosenthal, J. W., 7, 36
Ruanda spectacles, 128
saferty glasses, 93
Sàfilo, 126, 151
Salter, Gilbert, 38
Samco, 159
Sandra Deluxe, 141
Satan spectacles, 112
Schnaitman, Isaac, 33
scissors glasses, 26, 51
Sea Mist spectacle, 95, 98
Sears Roebuck and Co., 91, 107, 118
See Fair, 103
Selecta spectacles, 129
Sellers, Peter, 132, 154
shagreen case, 12, 19 28, 29, 74
sharkskin case, 11, 19, 20
Sharon spectacles, 108
shell case, 51
Sherman, 97
Shield rite lens, 113
shipping box, 50
Shuron Alum, 110, 116
Sibylle spectacles, 138
silver frame, 12, 14, 18, 20-26, 28-31, 39, 42-44, 53, 55, 57, 62, 71, 72, 105
sliding temple, 27, 29, 30-33
Smith, Addison, 18
snow goggles, 7, 64
So-easy eyeglasses, 62
Solar Spree spectacles, 160
Solomons, Elias, 30, 31
Space Odyssey spectacles, 134
Specialized glasses, 64-68

SRO, 109
star spectacles, 189
Statue of Liberty sunglasses, 190
steel bridge, 18
steel frames, 5, 17, 18, 20, 30, 31, 39, 51, 66, 68, 74, 78, 92
stereoscope picture, 50
Stokes, Henry, 66
Storks spectacles, 174
string earpiece, 12
Stuttgart, 60
sunglasses, 62, 65, 66, 69, 94-190
Sunmodes, 136, 155
supplementary lens, 93
Swank Optical eyewear, 116, 119, 135, 151, 159
Tamarin spectacles, 144
Taylor, C. W., 71
teastone lens, 12
temple spectacles, 17
temples, 2, 5, 12, 17, 37, 39, 51
Tennis Racquets spectacles, 170
tin case, 67, 93
TipTop sunglasses, 107
titanium, 185, 186
tortoiseshell case, 19, 37, 38, 51
tortoiseshell frame, 6, 11-16, 20, 21, 25, 27, 32, 37, 3383, 51, 57, 58, 62, 79, 80, 82-89
Trifari, 137
Tru-Vue, 115
Tura, Inc., 109, 130, 151
turnpin hinge, 18, 28
turtle, 37
tweezers, 21
Two Guitars spectacles, 170
Universal Optical Company, 114, 165
Variety-Libra, 163
Venice, Italy, 8
Villant, 113
Vous Gogo spectacles, 138
Wang, Vera Couture, 190
welder's goggles, 93, 94
Whitehouse, Walter W., 71
Whitney, 98
wig spectacles, 17, 18
Willson Goggles, 77
wiper blades spectacles, 189
wire frame, 39
wire temple, 39
wooden case, 13, 19, 22, 24, 39, 65
wooden frame, 7, 64, 65
x-bridge, 18, 39
Y-Not spectacles, 127
Yamada spectacles, 133
York, Pennsylvania, 79, 92
Zak spectacles, 136
Zig-zag spectacles, 185
Zylite, 109
Zyloware, 141

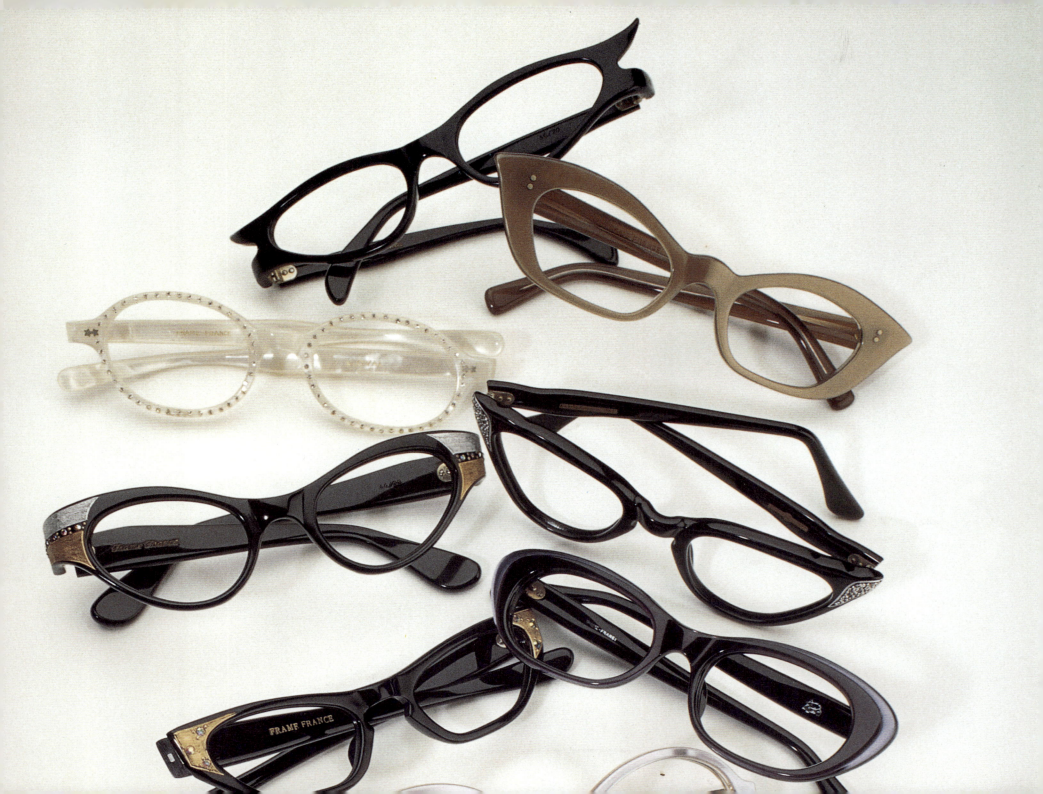